proach to

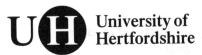

**University of
Hertfordshire**

College Lane, Hatfield, Herts. AL10 9AB

Learning and ~~~~~~ ~~~~~ .... 93) 785484 (Direct line)

Please return on or before the last date stamped below:

0 1 FEB 1999
0 9 DEC 1999
- 9 JUN 2000
- 4 APR 2001

WITHDRAWN

A Practical Approach to Breast Disease

Edited by

Lois F. O'Grady, M.D.

Professor of Medicine, University of
California, Davis, School of Medicine,
Davis; Attending Physician,
University of California, Davis,
Medical Center, Sacramento,
California

Karen K. Lindfors, M.D.

Associate Professor of Radiology,
University of California, Davis, School
of Medicine, Davis; Chief of Breast
Imaging, University of California,
Davis, Medical Center, Sacramento,
California

Lydia Pleotis Howell, M.D.

Associate Professor of Pathology,
University of California, Davis, School
of Medicine, Davis; Director of
Cytology, University of California,
Davis, Medical Center, Sacramento,
California

Mary B. Rippon, M.D.

Assistant Professor of Surgery,
University of California, Davis, School
of Medicine, Davis; Attending
Surgeon, University of California,
Davis, Medical Center, Sacramento,
California

ROYAL MILITARY COLLEGE OF SCIENCE
LIBRARY

Control No C3\663377 |

Class No.

Date Received   2 9 APR 1998

CL
616.
994
49
PRA

Little, Brown and Company
Boston   New York   Toronto   London

Copyright © 1995 by Lois F. O'Grady,
Karen K. Lindfors, Lydia Pleotis
Howell, and Mary B. Rippon

First Edition

All rights reserved. No part of this
book may be reproduced in any form
or by any electronic or mechanical
means, including information storage
and retrieval systems, without
permission in writing from the
publisher, except by a reviewer who
may quote brief passages in a review.

Library of Congress Cataloging-in-Publication Data

A Practical approach to breast disease / Lois F. O'Grady . . . [et al.].
    p. cm.
    Includes bibliographical references and index.
    ISBN 0-316-63377-1
    1. Breast—Diseases.   2. Breast—Cancer.   I. O'Grady, Lois F.
    [DNLM: 1. Breast Diseases—diagnosis.   2. Breast Diseases—
therapy.   WP 840 P895 1994]
    RG491.P73   1994
    616.99′449—dc20
    DNLM/DLC
    for Library of Congress   94-26205
                                               CIP

Printed in the United States of America

RRD-VA

Editorial: Nancy E. Chorpenning
Production Editor: Cathleen Cote
Copyeditor: Regina Knox
Indexer: Ann Blum
Production Supervisor: Louis C. Bruno, Jr.
Cover Designer: Michael A. Granger

To

The physicians of northern California
who have referred patients to us

The patients who have inspired us

The staff of the UC Davis Cancer
Center who have made it all possible

Contents

Contributing Authors

Margaret Deanesly, M.D.C.M.

Medical Director, Stanford Linear Accelerator Center, Palo Alto Medical Clinic, Menlo Park, California

Lydia Pleotis Howell, M.D.

Associate Professor of Pathology, University of California, Davis, School of Medicine, Davis; Director of Cytology, University of California, Davis, Medical Center, Sacramento, California

Virginia Joyce, M.D.

Attending Surgeon, University of California, Davis, Medical Center, Sacramento, California

Mary E. Kennedy, R.N., M.S.

Manager, Hospice Program, University of California, Davis, Medical Center, Sacramento, California

Karen K. Lindfors, M.D.

Associate Professor of Radiology, University of California, Davis, School of Medicine, Davis; Chief of Breast Imaging, University of California, Davis, Medical Center, Sacramento, California

Lois F. O'Grady, M.D.

Professor of Medicine, University of California, Davis, School of Medicine, Davis; Attending Physician, University of California, Davis, Medical Center, Sacramento, California

Richard H. Oi, M.D.

Professor of Obstetrics and Gynecology and of Pathology, University of California, Davis, School of Medicine; Attending Gynecologist, University of California, Davis, Medical Center, Sacramento, California

Linda Clemence Reib, B.S.

Certified Fitter; President, Enhance by Linda Reib and Co., Carmichael, California

Debra A. Reilly, M.D.

Assistant Professor of Plastic Surgery, University of California, Davis, School of Medicine, Davis; Attending Plastic Surgeon, University of California, Davis, Medical Center, Sacramento, California

Debra A. Reilly, M.D.   Assistant Professor of Plastic Surgery, University of California, Davis, School of Medicine, Davis; Attending Plastic Surgeon, University of California, Davis, Medical Center, Sacramento, California

Mary B. Rippon, M.D.   Assistant Professor of Surgery, University of California, Davis, School of Medicine, Davis; Attending Surgeon, University of California, Davis, Medical Center, Sacramento, California

Janice K. Ryu, M.D.   Assistant Professor of Radiation Therapy, University of California, Davis and San Francisco; Radiation Oncologist, University of California, Davis, Medical Center, Sacramento, California

Preface

The motivation behind *A Practical Approach to Breast Disease* came from two sources: our discussions with the physicians who have referred patients to us and our stimulating interaction as a multi-specialty team of physicians with a primary interest in breast diseases.

From our formal and informal consultations, it became obvious that many practitioners had a firm grasp of some of the information needed for the diagnosis and treatment of breast diseases, but gaps existed. The specialist-oriented literature did not provide an adequate framework with which the primary care physician could feel comfortable managing common problems, deciding what problems needed referral to the specialist, and providing follow-up care.

This book took shape as we listed the questions that we, as specialists in different aspects of breast diseases, were asked most frequently. The questions came up in patient referrals, in informal consultations, and in our weekly conference as we sat together discussing issues that needed clarification.

Our goal was the creation of a readable, succinct book on benign and malignant breast disease. It is oriented clinically with discussion of symptom complexes. It includes discussions of major aspects of patient care that are not strictly medical or surgical because we believe that too little attention has been directed toward these issues. We also have attempted to review controversial issues and advances, for example, the role of screening mammography in younger women and the pros and cons of adjuvant chemotherapy, so that the primary care physician can provide wise counsel. We have not addressed the details of chemotherapy nor the care of the patient with metastatic disease because these aspects of care are not usually within the purview of the primary care physician.

We have enjoyed writing this book and have learned much about each other's specialties. It is our desire that this knowledge is imparted to you in an interesting and informative way. We hope *A Practical Approach to Breast Disease* will find a favored place in your office and will enhance the care of all women with breast disease.

We would like to thank the American Cancer Society, California Division, for permission to adapt material from their pamphlet on breast self-examination. We appreciate the artistic talents of Nila Nilüfer Gönen, Fernando Herrera, and Donna Odle.

L. F. O.
K. K. L.
L. P. H.
M. B. R.

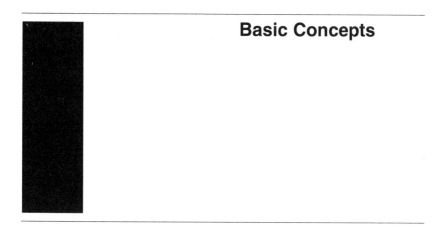

Basic Concepts

Notice. The indications and dosages of all drugs in this book have been recommended in the medical literature and conform to the practices of the general medical community. The medications described do not necessarily have specific approval by the Food and Drug Administration for use in the diseases and dosages for which they are recommended. The package insert for each drug should be consulted for use and dosage as approved by the FDA. Because standards for usage change, it is advisable to keep abreast of revised recommendations, particularly those concerning new drugs.

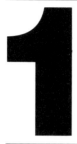

Anatomy and Physiology of the Adult Female Breast

Lydia Pleotis Howell

Common Questions

A basic understanding of anatomy and physiology is necessary for a full understanding of breast disease. Below are some common questions that physicians from various fields of medicine ask about the anatomy and physiology of the breast.

What are the normal anatomic variations in the female breast?
The adult female breast is not a well-delineated organ and varies in size, depending on the individual's body habitus, age, and menstrual cycle. The areola and nipple also vary in size and position. In general, the majority of the breast overlies the superior and medial portions of the pectoralis major, and is bordered by the clavicle and seventh costal cartilage above and below and the midline and margin of the latissimus dorsi medially and laterally. Breast parenchyma frequently extends into the axilla as the tail of Spence. The breast parenchyma is contained within the mammary adipose capsule, which gives the breast its smooth contour.

Supernumerary nipples and ectopic breast tissue can occur in areas other than the location described above and can be a source of benign and malignant breast tumors. Like all mammals, the human embryo develops a bilateral mammary ridge or milk line along the ventral aspect of the trunk from the axilla to the perineum. Although most sites other than those destined to become the breasts regress, beginning at 9 to 10 weeks of embryonic life, some of these areas may persist. Masses created by this tissue can be seen in the axilla and vulva in 1 to 2% of the population and can be the source of hidradenitis suppurativa in these locations. Supernumerary nipples are seen in 2.5% of neonates (with a slight male predominance) and typically resemble a nevus. Breast stroma and glands can be seen microscopically in the connective tissue below the supernumerary nipple.

What is the ligament of Cooper?
The ligament of Cooper, which is responsible for suspending the breast, is formed by the fusion of the pectoralis fascia with fibrous bands that extend from the superficial and deep fascial planes into

the breast parenchyma. The laxity of this structure that occurs with age causes ptotic breasts. Invasion of this ligament by cancer will shorten the breast and may cause the overlying skin to appear fixed.

How does the breast change with the menstrual cycle?
Patients frequently complain of breast discomfort at certain times during their menstrual cycle and breast examination can reveal simultaneous changing nodularity. Like the well-known morphologic changes that occur in the endometrium, microscopic changes in breast morphology also can be correlated to the menstrual cycle. These, however, are not prominent and are not noted by most pathologists on routine histologic examination.

During the endometrial proliferative phase that follows menstruation, the breast stroma is cellular and dense without edema, the lobules are simple, without secretions, and mitoses are absent. In the endometrial secretory phase, both the number and size of the mammary lobules increase. Vacuolated cells appear and become progressively more extensive, as does the presence of epithelial mitoses, stromal edema, and luminal secretions. Active apocrine secretion can also be seen late in this phase. During menstruation, epithelial degeneration and sloughing can be observed. The epithelial cells appear pyknotic with a loss of vacuolated cells so that eventually pale eosinophilic cells predominate. Mitoses decrease, and the stroma becomes more dense, metachromatic, with an abundant lymphocytic infiltrate.

How does the breast change with menopause?
Little is known about the factors that cause age-related atrophy of the breast, other than that it is related to estrogen and progesterone loss. After the age of 35, the breast loses some of its glandular component and lymphocytic infiltration occurs. This process accelerates at menopause with a marked reduction in the number of glands due to atrophy, fibrosis, and hyalinization. Atrophic cystic dilatation can occur in some lobules. Some terminal duct lobular units (TDLUs) persist and become hormonally autonomous, perhaps increasing the risk of breast cancer.

How does the breast change with pregnancy and lactation?
During pregnancy, the breasts grossly enlarge, develop a more noticeable vascular pattern, and the areola and nipple may darken. Microscopically, interlobular connective tissue and fat decrease, and glandular proliferation occurs, mainly in the first half of pregnancy. This is commonly referred to as adenosis or hyperplasia of pregnancy and consists of enlargement of existing lobules and formation of new ones. In the second half of pregnancy, proliferation slows and glandular differentiation is more prominent. The alveoli progressively dilate with secretions as the lining cells actively synthesize milk fat and cytoplasmic vacuolation becomes more conspicuous. This prese-

cretory function requires prolactin and is supported by insulin, human placental growth hormone, and glucocorticoids, but is partially inhibited by luteal and placental sex steroids such as progesterone. Following delivery, these antagonizing hormones are no longer present, and prolactin can exert its full effect so that lactation can occur. Suckling stimulates the release of both prolactin and adrenocorticotropic hormone, which maintains milk synthesis. Suckling also stimulates the release of oxytocin from the posterior pituitary for milk ejection.

The cessation of lactation with the concomitant decrease in prolactin levels leads to an involution of the breast that is caused by a poorly understood combination of mechanical, vascular, and hormonal influences. The glandular differentiation regresses to its prepregnancy state with fibrosis and hyalinization of many lobules and an increase in fat and connective tissue.

In what part of the breast does cancer arise?
Almost all benign and malignant breast pathology arises in the terminal duct lobular unit (TDLU) (Figs. 1-1 and 1-2). The lobes of the breast are composed of an arborized network of ducts. The distal terminus is the TDLU. Thousands of TDLUs form the functional secretory unit of the breast, whose product is drained through the branching ducts that lead to the ampullae at the surface of the nipple. The TDLU is a complex composed of the extralobular and intralobular terminal ducts and a cluster of ductules (acini). The ductules are lined by an inner layer of secretory cells and an outer layer of myoepithelial cells that contain contractile fibers that eject the milk into the ducts during lactation. The ductules plus the intralobular terminal duct constitute a lobule.

Do women with large breasts have more glandular elements and are they at greater risk for developing breast cancer?
Breast cancer risk is not based on the size of the breast. All female breasts, regardless of size, contain approximately the same number of lobes (15–25) that represent the glandular component of the breast. The variation in women's breast size is chiefly due to variations in the amount of connective tissue and fat in the breast. Larger breasts may be more difficult to examine clinically, so mammography is important to ensure the early discovery of breast cancer.

Why is the venous drainage of the breast important?
Breast cancer spreads via the veins in 50% of patients who develop metastases. Deep venous drainage is composed of three pathways: (1) the internal thoracic vein, which is the largest vein, (2) the axillary vein draining the chest wall and deep aspect of the breast, and (3) the intercostal veins. Each of these pathways leads to the pulmonary capillary network and represents a potential route for lung

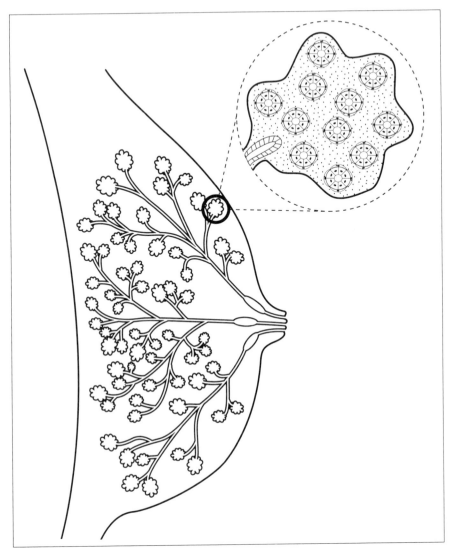

Fig. 1-1. The breast consists of a branching network of ducts that terminates at the terminal duct lobular unit *(inset)*, which is the site of origin for almost all pathologic conditions of the breast.

metastasis. In addition, because intercostal veins drain into the vertebral veins they also can provide a route for skeletal metastases.

What are the important sites of lymphatic drainage from the breast?
Breast cancer spreads by lymphatics in 20% of patients who develop metastases. The lymphatic drainage from the breast can be divided into various cutaneous and parenchymal channels. If the cutaneous lymphatics are obstructed by metastatic tumor, the characteristic peau d'orange appearance of the skin will result. The cutaneous lymphatics from the breast's lower border may also be the route for liver

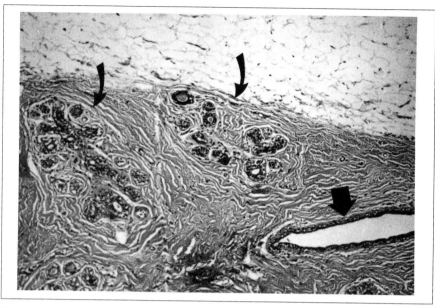

Fig. 1-2. Photomicrograph of the terminal duct lobular unit. Note that a slightly ectatic duct *(large arrow)* is leading to two lobules *(curved arrows)* (H&E, 100×).

metastases to occur because these drain directly into the epigastric plexus and then into the subdiaphragmatic and subperitoneal plexuses. The axilla receives the majority of the lymphatic drainage from the breast. There are three levels of nodes that are important to surgeons: level I, which is lateral to the pectoralis minor muscle; level II, which is under the pectoralis minor; and level III, which is medial to the pectoralis minor. Levels I and II receive the majority of the lymphatic drainage and are the most likely to be involved with metastases. Level III (the subclavicular group) represents the highest groups of nodes obtainable by surgical axillary dissection and receives the lymphatic drainage from all the other axillary nodes. Because they are not considered "regional" nodes their involvement is considered a poor prognostic sign.

Do benign breasts have detectable estrogen receptors?
Seven percent of the total breast epithelium is estrogen receptor–positive by microspectrophotometry and immunocytochemistry. These positive cells are scattered as single cells in the luminal surface or in the lobule wall. The breast stroma is estrogen receptor–negative on microspectrophotometry and immunocytochemistry.

Suggested Reading

Healey W, and Hodge W. *Surgical Anatomy.* Philadelphia: BC Decker, 1990. Pp. 42–51.

Jensen HM. Breast pathology, emphasizing precancerous and cancer-associated lesions. In RD Bulbrook and DJ Taylor (eds.), *Commentaries on Research in Breast Disease,* Vol. 2. New York: Alan R. Liss, 1981.

Longacre TA, and Bartow SA. A correlative morphologic study of human breast and endometrium in the menstrual cycle. *Am J Surg Pathol* 10:382–393, 1986.

McCarty KS, and Tucker JA. Breast. In S Sternberg (ed.), *Histology for Pathologists.* New York: Raven, 1992.

Petersen OW, Hower PE, and van Deurs B. Frequency and distribution of estrogen receptor-positive cells in normal, nonlactating human breast tissue. *J Natl Cancer Inst* 77:343–349, 1986.

Vogel PM, et al. The correlation of histologic changes in the human breast with the menstrual cycle. *Am J Pathol* 104:23–34, 1981.

Wellings SR, and Jensen HM. An atlas of subgross pathology of the human breast with special reference to possible precancerous lesions. *J Natl Cancer Inst* 55:231–273, 1975.

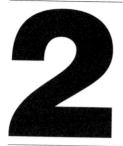

Nonmalignant Breast Disease

Lois F. O'Grady

Although there is an increasing incidence of breast cancer in the Western world, most breast lumps are benign. Over 75% of patients attending specialized breast disease clinics do so for nonmalignant breast disease. However, the media are rife with references to breast cancer, which increases concerns about breast health and prompts more women to seek evaluation of breast lumps and breast pain. All too often, once a cancer has been excluded, the woman's complaints are dismissed. The attitude is "After all, it's not cancer, so don't worry." Although this attitude may reflect a tendency to trivialize complaints of women, all too often it reflects the practitioner's lack of knowledge. Many of us have never been taught about nonmalignant breast disease, and the pertinent information is scattered in obscure places in the medical literature. This chapter provides a general review of nonmalignant disorders of the breast, addresses their relation, and considers their etiology.

The breast is designed to produce milk. Just as each menstrual cycle prepares the uterus for pregnancy, so does the cycle of hormone stimulation begin the changes that, in pregnancy, lead to milk production. Just as the uterine lining sloughs when pregnancy does not occur, so too does the stimulated breast tissue slough. The cellular debris is usually absorbed; sometimes it is extruded through the nipple as spontaneous secretions.

Sometimes the systems go awry: The normal ebb and flow becomes more pronounced or disordered; there is too much or too little of one of the stimulating hormones; the stimulation outstrips involution; the products of stimulation are not completely reabsorbed; normal structure becomes disordered; or lumps and bumps, which are sometimes painful, occur.

In trying to make some sense of the disorders of the breast, it is helpful to consider them in three parts (Table 2-1): (1) disorders of the entire breast, irrespective of anatomy, such as trauma or infection, (2) disorders of the major ducts, such as galactorrhea or papilloma, and (3) disorders of the terminal duct lobular unit (TDLU), such as fibrocystic disease.

Table 2-1. Benign conditions of the female breast

Disorders of entire breast	Disorders of major ducts	Disorders of the TDLU
Trauma	Galactorrhea	Fibrocystic disease
Hematoma	Galactocele	Adenosis (sclerosing
Ruptured cyst	Mammary duct ectasia	adenosis)
Fat necrosis	(comedomastitis)	Cystic disease
Infection	Papilloma	Hyperplasia
		Fibroadenomata

TDLU = terminal duct lobular unit.

Disorders of the Entire Breast

Trauma

Lying on the anterior chest, the breast is an easy target for trauma. Just as a patient often is unable to tell which bump produced which bruise on the hand or forearm because they occur so frequently, busy and active women sometimes do not recall the trauma that set off a symptom complex in the breast.

Trauma can lead to any one of, or combination of, three conditions: (1) hematoma, (2) ruptured cyst, or (3) fat necrosis. All three can present with the sudden onset of pain or discomfort and it may be impossible to distinguish them clinically. There may or may not be a mass or discoloration, depending on how deep in the breast the lesion lies. Some clinical clues to distinguishing the conditions exist: hematomas tend to cause discoloration; ruptured cysts tend to occur in women with a history of cystic disease; and fat necrosis tends to occur in women with pendulous breasts, tends to cause erythema, and the resultant scarring can cause nipple retraction. An example of hematoma with fat necrosis is seen in Fig. 2-1. The treatment is symptomatic.

It is permissible to watch the patient with evidence of trauma over the course of 4 to 6 weeks. But, if at the end of 4 to 6 weeks there is still a mass and/or discoloration, it *must* be investigated with mammography and possibly with needle aspiration or surgical biopsy.

Infection

Infection, with its concomitant erythema, soreness, and mass effect, is usually self-evident. Small areas of infection can be treated with oral antibiotics, but larger areas require intravenous antibiotics for a day or two before oral administration. Organisms are usually gram-positive, and antibiotics should be chosen with this in mind. Suspected areas of abscess formation should be drained.

Infection occurs primarily in nursing women. It is very unusual in

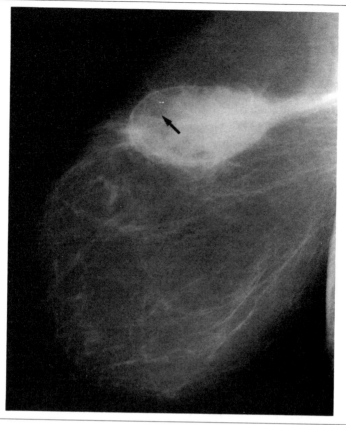

Fig. 2-1. Hematoma with fat necrosis. A large ill-defined hematoma is noted in the superior right breast on this mediolateral oblique view. The patient has an ecchymotic area in the overlying skin. She reported recent trauma to her breast. The mass showed partial resolution on a subsequent mammogram. Note also the more lucent area *(arrow)* within the hematoma; this represents fat necrosis resulting from the trauma.

a nonnursing woman. *An abscess or major breast infection in a nonnursing woman raises a red flag, because it can be confused with inflammatory cancer.* If the infection does not clear readily, it should be incised, cultured, and drained. If an abscess is present, the wall of the cavity should be biopsied to look for an underlying malignancy.

Disorders of the Major Ducts

Disorders of the major ducts are grouped together because they are anatomically similar and because they present with nipple discharge (see Chap. 9). Nipple discharge is not uncommon. Up to 20% of women may have a few drops of milky, opalescent, or clear fluid appear spontaneously or on palpation. In these women breast manipulation or suckling may be an integral part of sexual activity.

The discharge is small and unchanged over years. It may occur during the menses as the premenstrual hyperplastic changes involute.

Galactorrhea

When the amount of fluid increases beyond a drop or two, the term *galactorrhea* is used. It is critical to note whether the discharge is from multiple ducts, which tends to be of benign etiology, or from a single duct, which could reflect an underlying malignancy.

There are three basic causes of galactorrhea (Table 2-2). First, *excessive stimulation* from sexual activity or from running or jogging without a support bra can cause the disorder. If the milk is noted to come from multiple ducts on the nipple and ceases or decreases with temporary cessation of the activity, nothing more need be done because it is a physiologic response. Second, there are large numbers of *drugs* that can induce galactorrhea (see Table 2-2), all by a common pathway of hyperprolactinemia. A history of recent drug use, and a cessation of galactorrhea when the drug is temporarily discontinued confirm that it is of benign nature. Mammography is not indicated. The third and most worrisome cause are *hypothalamic-pituitary disorders.* New-onset galactorrhea, especially if accompanied by menstrual abnormalities and no drug history, requires investigation. Serum prolactin levels as well as radiologic investigation of the chest (occasionally a bronchogenic carcinoma secretes prolactin) and of the sella turcica (for possibility of pituitary adenoma) may be performed before an endocrinologist is consulted.

Galactocele

Seen only in nursing or recently nursing women, galatocele is a large, milk-filled cyst that forms a palpable mass in the breast. It may be soft or may feel rock-hard. If it occurs suddenly, it may cause acute pain. Galactocele is treated readily with simple needle aspiration, but if it recurs biopsy may be warranted to rule out underlying pathology.

Mammary Duct Ectasia (Comedomastitis)

In some women, a few (always more than one, rarely all) of the major ducts are subject to repeated episodes of periductal inflammation. The resultant scarring leads to distortion, thickening, and widening of the ducts near the areola. The exact etiology is unknown. It tends to occur in multiparous older women. During periods of inflammation anaerobic bacteria are found, which are different from the usual organisms in the typical lactational cellulitis/abscess that are aerobic gram-positive. The patient typically notes secretion of a thick cheesy material (it is in fact cheese) from the affected ducts. In addition, the patients have one or more of the following: noncyclic mas-

Table 2-2. Causes of galactorrhea

Mechanical stimulation of the nipple
Drugs
   Estrogenic
     Digitalis
     Marijuana
     Heroin
     Dopamine receptor blockers
     Phenothiazines
     Haloperidol
     Metoclopramide
     Isoniazid
   Dopamine depleters
     Tricyclic antidepressants
     Reserpine
     Methyldopa
     Cimetidine
     Bendodiazepines
Hypothalamic-pituitary disorders

talgia, nipple retraction, subareolar breast lump, inflammatory changes in and around the nipple-areolar complex, or periareolar abscess with or without fistula.

Mammography may show prominent ducts under the areola (Fig. 2-2) and characteristic periductal calcifications, but is not often diagnostic. Mild disease may respond to intermittent antibiotic usage (be sure the antibiotic chosen is effective against anaerobes), but most patients require surgical excision of the affected ducts. Duct ectasia is benign and is not associated with malignancy.

Papilloma

Papillomas can occur anywhere along the ductal structure, but the solitary ones, which are more common, tend to occur near the nipple. Figure 2-3 shows an artist's sketch of a cross section of a breast with the nipple-areolar complex progressively enlarged. A duct near the nipple is magnified to show a papilloma. In Fig. 2-3D, the papilloma can be seen on a stalk, producing its characteristic secretion of serous or bloody fluid that is often secreted at the nipple. *Papillomas, like cancers that cause a nipple discharge, produce a discharge from one duct and one duct only. This is a major diagnostic point.* On questioning, the patient will report that the secretion is always at the same point on the nipple. This single-duct secretion can usually be confirmed by milking the duct on examination, and is enough to send the patient directly to the surgeon. It is possible to perform galactography to visualize the papilloma and pinpoint its location. However, its use is controversial; many surgeons prefer to cannulate the duct with fine wire or plastic to guide the excision.

Papillomas can become large enough to be palpable or to appear

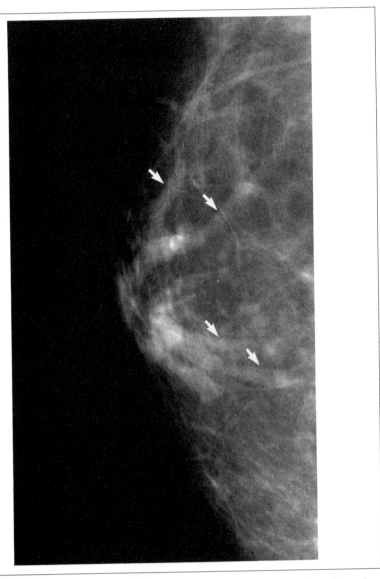

Fig. 2-2. Duct ectasia. Multiple ectatic ducts *(arrows)* are seen in the subareolar area on this craniocaudal mammogram.

on mammogram. Occasionally, they can be seen on ultrasonograms of the breast (Fig. 2-4). Cytologic examination of the discharge is only helpful if positive. Because the usual recommendation is to excise the lesion to rule out cancer and to prevent malignancy (fortunately not common with solitary papillomas), one can proceed directly to surgery.

Multiple papillomas can present in the same way. They are less common, tend to occur more peripherally, and have a much higher incidence of malignant degeneration.

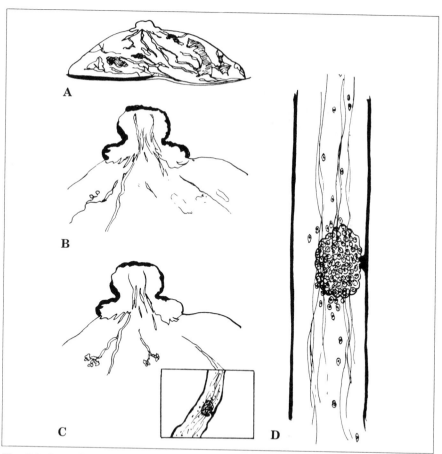

Fig. 2-3. Intraductal papilloma. An artist's drawing of a subgross section of a breast with the nipple complex progressively enlarged (A through D) to show a duct near the nipple with a papilloma on a stalk, and weeping cellular and serosanguineous debris.

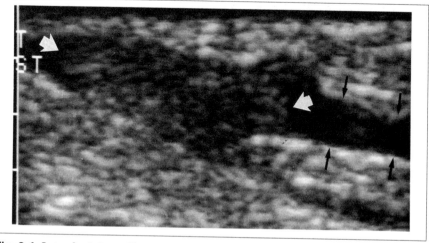

Fig. 2-4. Intraductal papilloma. An ultrasound of the left breast oriented along the course of a dilated duct *(black arrows)* that had been visualized mammographically. A 2.5-cm solid mass *(white arrows)* is located within the duct; histologic examination revealed an intraductal papilloma.

Disorders of the Terminal Duct Lobular Unit

Fibrocystic Disease

The normal breast consists of a series of terminal ducts with their associated lobular units (TDLUs), dispersed in a fibro-fatty stroma. These TDLUs are subject to monthly cycles of stimulation and growth as well as withdrawal of stimulation and resultant involution. When the breast is stimulated and full, there is nodularity to the breast and sometimes discomfort; when it is involuted it is softer, less nodular, and not tender.

As in all things, there is a spectrum of normalcy. Some breasts have no nodularity, some a great deal. Some breasts are never tender, some are always painful. When the changes are extreme, they call attention to themselves—they are recognized as "abnormal," and we call them disease. Unfortunately, these extreme changes were given, years ago, the title of fibrocystic *disease* and were subcategorized by whether there was primarily stromal proliferation (fibrosis), glandular proliferation (adenosis), both (sclerosing adenosis), or cystic formation (cystic disease). The problems with this classification are that (1) patients with clinical mastalgia and nodularity may have neither fibrosis nor cyst formation and (2) the different elements may predominate in different areas of the breast. In addition, mild forms of the disorder occur often enough in women that it is not necessarily a "disease."

Based on the physiologic background of the syndrome, the Welsh have coined the phrase ANDI—**a**bnormality of **n**ormal **d**evelopment and **i**nvolution. It is more apt than *fibrocystic disease,* but it is difficult to change terminology that is entrenched. The term benign breast disorder (BBD) is often used, but there are other breast disorders (e.g., mastititis, fibroadenoma) that are benign and are *not* part of the fibrocystic symptom complex.

Pathophysiology

Pathologically, excessive stimulation of the breast may lead to hyperplastic lobules, and lack of complete involution with each menstrual cycle may lead to accumulation of cells in the lobule (Fig. 2-5A). Sometimes the cellular debris may not be completely reabsorbed, leaving a full, tense lobule. In some women, hyperplastic changes in the ducts may impede drainage. With time the lobule may distend with cells and/or debris. The distention of one lobule may induce torsion of its duct or an adjacent one, preventing complete drainage of debris from the duct. With time a small cyst evolves, then two cysts may merge, and the cysts may become large (see Fig. 2-5) and tense. If a cyst ruptures, inflammation ensues, as does a fibrotic reaction. If a biopsy is done, the pathologist sees a spectrum of normal to very hyperplastic lobules, a spectrum of dilated lobules to macrocysts, and perhaps areas of fibrosis.

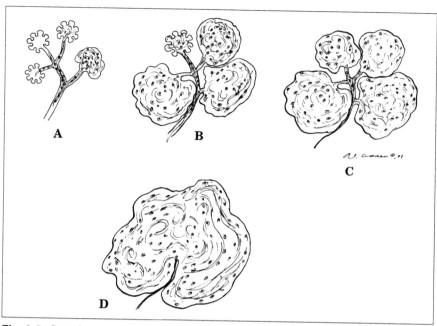

Fig. 2-5. Cyst formation. A. A terminal ductal-lobular unit is shown with one lobule distended with debris. As other lobules become distended (B, C), the entire group evolves into a large cyst (D).

The cystic changes themselves are not considered premalignant. However, there does seem to be an increased incidence of cancer in women with florid cystic disease. The malignant potential lies in the ductal hyperplasia that distorts or blocks the duct, leading to the cyst formation.

The proliferative changes are usually benign, but in 4 to 5% of patients the cells lining the ducts are atypical. It is these patients who are at increased risk of developing an invasive cancer. Unless a biopsy happens to be done to evaluate a mass or mammographic change, the clinician never knows whether a patient with fibrocystic changes has atypical hyperplasia or just hyperplasia. It is wise to have increased suspicion of malignancy in all patients with fibrocystic changes unless, for some reason, a biopsy is done and it becomes certain that the breast harbors no atypical changes.

Clinical Picture

Clinically, the fibrocystic disorder is manifested by palpable breast masses which are usually associated with an uncomfortable sense of tension and pain in the breast. The size of the masses and the degree of discomfort fluctuate with the menstrual cycle—being worse just before the menstrual bleed. The number and size of the masses as well as the degree of discomfort tend to progress until menopause when endogenous estrogen production decreases. Postmenopausal estrogen replacement may prolong the symptoms.

The pain may or may not be cyclic (see Chap. 8). Fibrocystic changes usually produce cyclic pain, but in its more severe form it is present continually. Noncyclic pain is more likely secondary to ductal ectasia or musculoskeletal diseases. It is important to document that the pain originates in the breast and not in the chest wall. Examination with the patient leaning forward with the breast falling away from the chest is helpful. The cyclic nature should be evident by history. If the patient is unsure, it might be helpful if she keeps a calendar of symptoms for a month or two.

The nodularity is usually bilateral and concentrated in the lateral quadrants of the breast, particularly in the upper, outer quadrant. Masses may be flat and platelike; or they may feel like peas, BB shot, or discrete round masses. Cysts may be soft, rock-hard, or anywhere in between. As one palpates an area of nodularity one feels for a discrete, dominant mass that is different from anything else in the breast and that may represent malignancy. Very often, fibrocystic changes disperse into strands under gentle palpation, cancers do not. *But no one has a microscope in their fingertips: only a biopsy can confirm the benignity of a discrete mass* (see Chaps. 5 and 7).

Fibroadenoma

These are benign tumors usually affecting women in their teens and twenties. They usually present as a solitary, firm mass, freely moveable in the breast, with a distinct, characteristic picture mammo-

Fig. 2-6. Fibroadenoma. Classic fibroadenoma that appears as a well-circumscribed lobulated mass containing coarse benign calcifications.

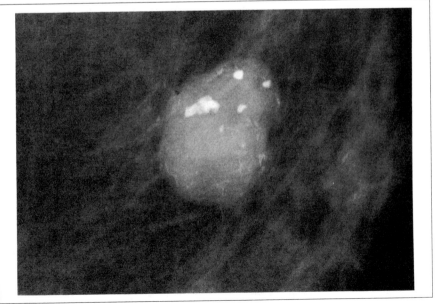

graphically (Fig. 2-6). Multiple fibroadenomas occasionally are seen. The lesions are considered an abnormality of normal development and involution rather than a tumor—an exuberant overgrowth of elements of the TDLU. One can look upon it as an extreme example of a hyperplastic lobule. Fibroadenomas rarely become malignant. They are considered here to separate them firmly from any association with fibrocystic disease.

Diagnosis of fibroadenoma is made easily with fine needle aspirates (provided experienced cytopathologists are available) or biopsy. Because they are quite characteristic and occur typically in young women, mammography is not always performed. Most are removed, but more for cosmetic and emotional reasons than for medical necessity. In postmenopausal women not on replacement estrogen, a fine needle diagnosis of fibroadenoma should correlate well with the clinical picture and mammogram. If it does not, or if the suspect fibroadenoma increases in size, excisional biopsy should be done to exclude phyllodes tumor.

Evaluation of the Patient with Mastalgia and Nodularity

Step one in the evaluation of the patient with mastalgia and nodularity is to obtain a general history and to perform an examination to exclude any underlying disease. Step two is a thorough examination of the breasts, with careful notation of nodular areas. This is a good time to teach the patient breast self-examination (see Appendix A).

If a dominant mass is identified, it must be completely evaluated (see Chap. 7). In women over the age of 30, mammography should be performed to assess the characteristics of the mass and to screen the rest of the breast tissue for associated abnormalities. Occasionally, fibrocystic disease can produce spiculated lesions that radiologists interpret as *radial scars* or *complex sclerosing lesions*. These may require biopsy to exclude carcinoma.

Mammography should be performed before any intervention for two reasons: (1) Hematomas caused by fine needle aspiration (FNA) or core needle biopsies may confound mammographic interpretation. Hematomas frequently look like ill-defined masses and thus can be confused with cancers on mammography. (2) On rare occasions, mammography may demonstrate a lesion with unequivocally benign characteristics, such as a calcified fibroadenoma or a lipoma with its typical fat-density, and diagnostic intervention can be avoided. Ultrasound can tell whether a mass is cystic or solid, but is not necessary if the mass is to be aspirated; the aspirator will easily discover whether it is cystic or not.

After mammography has been performed, most patients with dominant masses will undergo *FNA,* which will provide the diagnosis in solid lesions and will be diagnostic and therapeutic if the lesion is a cyst. If a cyst is aspirated and disappears completely, the area should be rechecked by physical examination in 3 months. Residual or recurrent masses need to be biopsied.

Even if no mass has been visualized on the mammogram, FNA should be performed on patients with dominant masses. Mammography has a false-negative rate of about 10%. One of the most frequent causes of malpractice litigation in breast cancer patients is delay in diagnosis when a practitioner assumes a mass is "OK" because it is not seen on the mammogram.

If a cytopathologist is not available for performance and interpretation of FNA, then core needle biopsy or excisional biopsy may be performed on a dominant mass. The biopsy material *must* be sent fresh to pathology, never in fixative, so that the pathologist can process the material appropriately to determine hormone receptors and tumor markers.

In women under the age of 30 with palpable masses, mammography must be used judiciously. This more cautious approach is based on data from atomic bomb survivors, from women exposed to repeated fluoroscopy, and from women treated with radiation for Hodgkin's disease, which show that the young breast may be at increased risk for breast cancer if it is exposed to excessive radiation. Most palpable masses in this age group will not prove to be cancer, and it is often possible to avoid imaging altogether and to proceed directly to FNA. If imaging studies are desired to confirm the presence of a mass in a young woman, ultrasound is generally performed first. If ultrasound is inconclusive, a limited mammogram may be performed to look for calcifications. Mammography should not be performed in women under the age of 20.

If a patient under 30 years of age does prove to have a malignant lesion, mammography can be performed subsequently. The radiologist will not be able to optimally assess the area in which the FNA was performed, but the assessment of surrounding and contralateral tissues for other lesions will not be compromised.

Once the physician and the patient are satisfied that there is no malignancy present in the patient with mastalgia and nodularity, therapeutic intervention, usually hormonal manipulation, may be considered (see Chap. 8).

Benign Disorders of the Male Breast

Gynecomastia

Men also can develop benign breast conditions as well as breast cancer. The male breast contains ductal structures, but no lobular tissue, and is not subject to cyclic hormonal stimulation. However, under the influence of excessive estrogen stimulation, the ductal

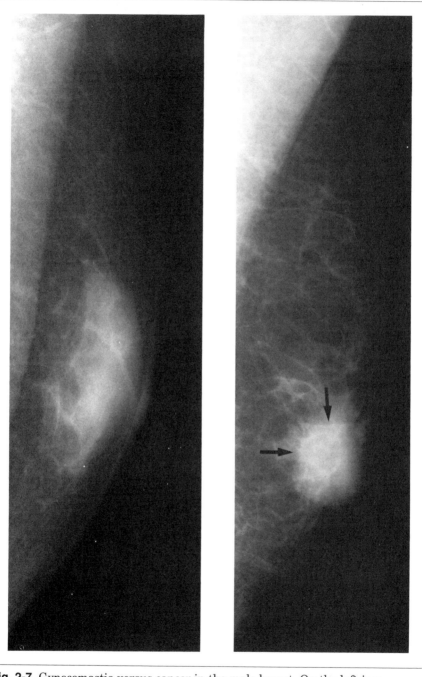

Fig. 2-7. Gynecomastia versus cancer in the male breast. On the left is a mediolateral view of the left breast in a male with gynecomastia. There is a flame-shaped or triangular area of architecturally normal appearing glandular tissue deep to the nipple. On the right is a mediolateral view of the left breast in a male with breast cancer. Note the ill-defined, high-density mass with convex borders *(arrows)* in the subareolar area.

structures and stroma can hypertrophy and lead to gynecomastia. This condition usually is seen at puberty. Forty percent of boys will have some degree of gynecomastia for a year or two until androgen production increases. After the age of 60, when androgen production begins to fall off, there is an increasing incidence (as much as 30%) of gynecomastia.

Many drugs induce gynecomastia. Interestingly, the drugs are the same as those that produce galactorrhea in women (see Table 2-2) with the addition of spironolactone and steroid hormones with estrogenic activity. Any condition that decreases androgen production (e.g., cryptorchidism, Klinefelter's syndrome) or increases estrogen (e.g., liver disease, starvation refeeding, tumors) can lead to gynecomastia.

Examination of the patient with gynecomastia shows a firm disk of often tender retroareolar tissue. Gynecomastia is more often bilateral than unilateral, although often asymmetric. Unilateral disease increases the suspicion of malignancy. Mammography can often distinguish the two (Fig. 2-7) and FNA is diagnostic for either.

Suggested Reading

Braunstein GD. Gynecomastia. *N Engl J Med* 328:490–495, 1993.

Drukker BH, and deMendonca WC. Fibrocystic changes and fibrocystic disease of the breast. *Obstet Gynecol Clin North Am* 14:685–702, 1987.

Hughes LE, Mansel RE, and Webster DJT. Nipple discharge. In *Benign Disorders and Diseases of the Breast*. London: Bailliere-Tindall, 1989. pp. 133–142.

Jensen HM. Breast pathology, emphasizing precancerous and cancer–associated lesions. *Commentaries on Research in Breast Disease* 2:41–86, 1981.

Longacre TA, and Bartow SA. A correlative morphologic study of human breast and endometrium in the menstrual cycle. *Am J Surg Pathol* 10(6):382–393, 1986.

Page DL, et al. Atypical hyperplastic lesions of the female breast. *Cancer* 55:2698–2708, 1985.

Sismondi P, et al. Benign breast disease: An update. *Clin Exp Obstet Gynecol* (Padova) 17:57–116, 1990.

Vorherr H. Fibrocystic breast disease: Pathophysiology, pathomorphology, clinical picture, and management. *Am J Obstet Gynecol* 154:161–179, 1986.

Webster DJT. Benign disorders of the male breast. *World J Surg* 13:726–730, 1989.

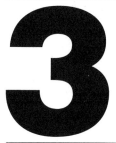

The Pathway to Cancer

Lydia Pleotis Howell

The etiology of breast cancer is as yet unknown. However, many factors are known to increase the risk for the development of the disease (Table 3-1). This chapter discusses the environmental, genetic, and morphologic changes that may be involved. In addition, the morphologic features of the various types of breast cancer and their clinical significance are discussed.

Environmental Factors

Diet

The role of diet in the development of breast cancer remains controversial. Many studies have examined the relationship between dietary fat and breast cancer. These studies have been prompted by the observation that breast cancer is a major killer of women in countries with high-fat diets, while its incidence is a lesser problem in Asian countries and others in which a lower amount of dietary fat is consumed. Interestingly, the incidence of breast cancer in Japan has risen as their diet has become more Westernized. Diet is only one variable among many lifestyle differences that may be important when comparing cancer incidence in various parts of the world. Genetics and other unidentified environmental differences may also play a role.

Comparison of studies on the role of diet tend to be contradictory. Goodwin and Boyd reviewed international correlation studies that consistently demonstrated a strong positive correlation between breast cancer and dietary fat. But when stronger case-controlled study designs with cohorts were used, a significant association between cancer and dietary fat could not be consistently demonstrated. Howe and colleagues' review of 12 case-controlled studies found a positive correlation between breast cancer risk and saturated fat intake in postmenopausal women. Vitamin C, and fruit and vegetable consumption were also considered to be important dietary factors. Other recent studies, including the National Health and Nutrition Examination Survey I, have shown no significant relationship between dietary fat and breast cancer. The role of diet continues to be controversial and will be examined as part of the National

Table 3-1. High-risk factors for breast cancer

Age: Older
Race: White
Age at birth of first child: 30+
Postmenopausal body build: Obese
Age at menarche: Early
Age at menopause: Late
Family history of breast cancer: First-degree relative, especially
    premenopausal bilateral breast cancer
History of breast disease: Atypical hyperplasia, previous breast cancer in
    one breast
History of other cancers: Ovarian or endometrial cancer

Women's Health Initiative which was funded by Congress in 1993 and is currently under way.

Hormonal Environment: Menarche, Menopause, and Childbearing

A woman's own hormonal environment may be a more important factor than diet in considering her risk for developing breast cancer. Early onset of menarche, late menopause, and late age at first pregnancy have all been shown to increase breast cancer risk. Early menarche and late menopause may also be related to nutrition because they occur with greatest frequency in prosperous, well-nourished countries. Both contribute to long-term, uninterrupted cyclical hormonal stimulation of the breast. As discussed in Chap. 1, the breast epithelium undergoes proliferation and regression with each menstrual cycle; such long-term repetitive stimulation may potentiate the development of malignant cells that escape the cycle and grow without restraint. Likewise, women who have had oophorectomies early in life rarely have breast cancer because they do not experience the cyclical alterations associated with ovulation. Obese postmenopausal women have an increased risk of breast cancer because fat is involved with estrogen production, creating a hyperestrogenic state and prolonged, uninterrupted hormonal stimulation of the breast.

Genetic Factors

As many as 31% of women treated for breast cancer at Memorial Sloan-Kettering Cancer Center report having at least one female relative with the same disease. While many of these represent sporadic and not genetically related cases, family history can increase a woman's risk of breast cancer. A woman with a first-degree relative (i.e., mother, sister, or daughter) with breast cancer has a 2.3 times greater relative risk of developing breast cancer; with a second-degree relative (e.g., grandmother, aunt) with breast cancer the relative risk is 1.5 times greater. If a woman has both a mother and a sister with breast cancer, her relative risk is 14 times greater. Risk is also increased if the relative's breast cancer was detected at a young age. No particular histologic type of breast cancer is consistently associated with family history in all classes of relatives. However, maternal breast cancer is more frequent in women with medullary carcinoma, and patients with lobular carcinoma more frequently have a sister with carcinoma.

Recently, a *breast cancer susceptibility gene, BRCA1,* has been identified on chromosome 17 and appears to be involved in approximately 5% of all breast cancers. This represents an inherited form of the disease and is manifest in families with multiple members who develop breast cancer at an early age. BRCA1 is located in the same area as other genes, such as Her-2-Neu, that are known to be involved in breast cancer. The Her-2-Neu gene correlates with a shorter time to relapse and disease-free survival when this gene's product is overexpressed. BRCA1 has been found to cause most of the inherited breast and ovarian cancer combinations. However, only 45% of families with breast cancer appear to be linked to this gene. Other as yet unknown mechanisms, possibly including other genes, and chance are most likely factors in the other 55% of cases.

Morphologic Precursors to Invasive Breast Cancer

The terminal duct lobular unit (TDLU), as described in Chap. 1, is the site of origin for almost all breast pathology, both benign and malignant. The benign condition of the breast that is commonly known as fibrocystic disease (see Chap. 2) is actually a spectrum of morphologic changes in the TDLU, many of which result from cellular proliferation (hyperplasia). Each of these changes has a different relative risk for development of breast cancer (Table 3-2). It is

Table 3-2. Breast lesions and relative risk for invasive breast cancer

No increased risk	Slightly increased risk (1.5–2.0×)	Moderately increased risk (5×)	Markedly increased risk (10×)
Adenosis	Hyperplasia	Atypical	Carcinoma in
Apocrine	(moderate or	hyperplasia	situ
metaplasia	florid, solid or	(ductal or	Atypical
Cysts	papillary)	lobular)	hyperplasia
Duct ectasia	Papillomatosis		with family
Fibroadenoma			history of
Fibrosis			breast cancer
Hyperplasia, mild			
Mastitis			
Squamous			
metaplasia			

as yet unclear if this morphologic continuum is also a biologic pre-neoplastic continuum because the natural history of these lesions is unknown. When these lesions are noted pathologically, it is best to consider them in the context of their associated risk.

Histologic Changes

No Increased Risk

Figures 3-1 and 3-2 illustrate the histologic changes that do not denote any increased risk for the development of invasive breast cancer. These typical fibrocystic changes usually occur in combination and include the following: (1) *adenosis,* a benign proliferation of acini within a lobule that can also be referred to as *sclerosing adenosis* when associated with fibrosis and distortion of the lobule; (2) *apocrine metaplasia,* a change in which the epithelium of the TDLU resembles those of apocrine sweat glands by gaining cytoplasm that is more abundant, pink, and granular, and is often associated with *cysts* of various sizes (see Fig. 3-2); (3) *duct ectasia,* a dilatation of medium-to-large ducts lined by flattened cells, filled with amorphous debris, and associated with periductal inflammation; and (4) *fibrosis.* *Epithelial hyperplasia* represents a spectrum of complexity in the proliferation of cells lining the TDLU, both quantitatively and qualitatively. In *mild hyperplasia,* there are not many more cells beyond the normal two-cell layer, and the cells do not have any significant nuclear changes.

Another benign breast lesion that is not part of the spectrum of fibrocystic changes, but which also arises in the TDLU, is *fibroadenoma* (Fig. 3-3) (see Chap. 2, Fig. 2-6). These do not increase the risk

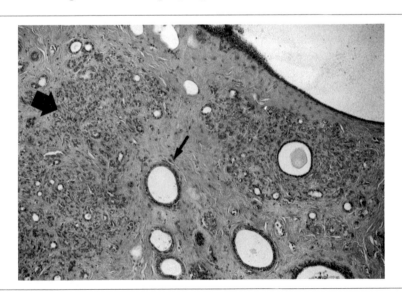

Fig. 3-1. Fibrocystic changes. Large arrow indicates area of adenosis. Small area in upper-right corner illustrates part of a large cyst. Note the fibrous stroma (H&E, 100×).

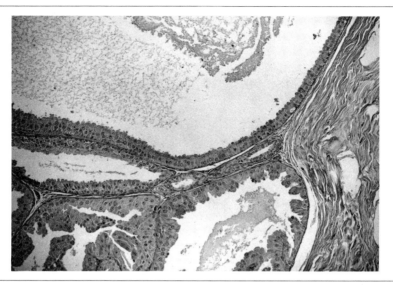

Fig. 3-2. Cysts lined by cells that have undergone apocrine metaplasia. Note that the lining cells are not flattened as in the cysts shown in Fig. 3-1, but instead are lined by larger cells with more abundant granular cytoplasm (H&E, 250×).

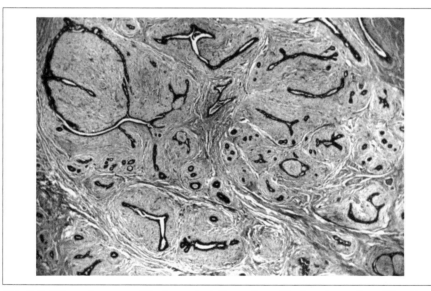

Fig. 3-3. Fibroadenoma with characteristic pericanalicular stromal proliferation compressing glands into slits (H&E, 100×).

of invasive breast cancer, though they have been noted on rare occasions to harbor in situ lobular carcinomas.

Slightly Increased Risk (1.5–2.0 Times)

Moderate or florid hyperplasia (sometimes referred to as usual-type hyperplasia) (Figs. 3-4 and 3-5A) is found in 20% of breast biopsies.

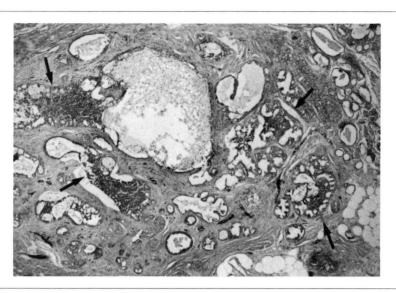

Fig. 3-4. Moderate hyperplasia without atypia. Note that in addition to fibrosis and cysts, there is more epithelial proliferation within the ductal spaces *(arrows)* (H&E, 100×).

This proliferative process usually involves more than five cell layers that distend the space. The cells vary in appearance and lack the monotonous appearance characteristic of malignant cells. They maintain their parallel, polarized, or swirling orientation and form irregular, slitlike spaces, unlike the rigidity round spaces in the classical cribriform pattern of ductal carcinoma in situ. *Papillomas* are frondlike or fingerlike growths with a fibrovascular core. There is always associated epithelial hyperplasia of varying degrees. Papillomas can occur in large or small ducts and can be solitary or multiple. When multiple and small, the term *papillomatosis* is used.

Moderately Increased Risk (5 Times)

This important category includes two forms of epithelial hyperplasia: atypical ductal hyperplasia and atypical lobular hyperplasia. Both of these lesions originate in the TDLU, and their designation as ductal or lobular indicates an aspect of their microscopic pattern rather than their site of origin. These lesions are characterized microscopically by having many, but not all, of the histologic features of car-

Fig. 3-5. Usual-type hyperplasia, atypical hyperplasia, and cribriform hyperplasia can closely resemble one another and can be difficult to distinguish. A. An enlargement of a hyperplastic area from Fig. 3-4. The spaces formed by the epithelial proliferation create irregularly shaped spaces and differ from the round, rigid spaces lined by monotonous cells that characterize the cribriform ductal carcinoma in situ shown in (B). Atypical ductal hyperplasia (C) has features intermediate between the two. Note that the nuclei do not appear as monotonous and not all the spaces appear rigid (H&E, 250×).

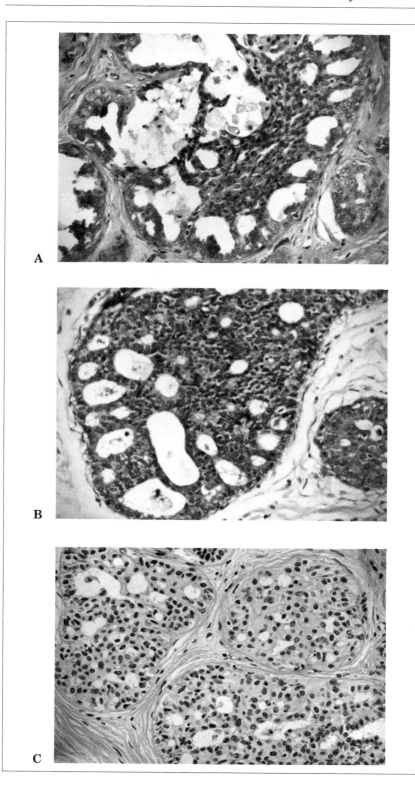

cinoma in situ, and therefore are often difficult for pathologists to diagnose. Studies have shown a lack of interobserver reproducibility, even among expert breast pathologists, in categorizing these proliferative lesions. However, if standardized diagnostic criteria are strictly followed, interobserver concordance should be quite high. When in doubt between a diagnosis of atypical hyperplasia and carcinoma in situ, pathologists should choose the more benign designation.

ATYPICAL DUCTAL HYPERPLASIA (ADH) (Fig. 3-5C) is characterized by a population of evenly spaced, uniform cells with monotonous hyperchromatic nuclear features, similar to those seen in ductal carcinoma in situ (DCIS). These cells may form the rigid geometric structures also seen in DCIS, but these atypical cells only involve part of the membrane-bound ductal-lobular space.

ATYPICAL LOBULAR HYPERPLASIA (ALH) is characterized by a population of bland, round cells that are evenly spaced and are often of smaller size than those seen in ADH or DCIS. These cells resemble those of lobular carcinoma in situ, but do not completely fill and distend the acinus, leaving intercellular spaces; less than half of the multiple acini in a lobular unit are involved.

Markedly Increased Risk (10 Times)

Carcinoma in situ is considered to be a true precursor to invasive breast cancer because it is often noted in and around invasive cancers and because invasive cancer often develops if these lesions are incompletely excised. Carcinoma in situ is typically divided into two major types: ductal and lobular (Table 3-3). Like the designation for atypical hyperplasia, these terms denote a histologic pattern and do not indicate the site of origin—all arise in the TDLU.

DUCTAL CARCINOMA IN SITU. There are numerous pathologic subdivisions for DCIS that are chiefly descriptive and are not used uniformly by all pathologists. The most important clinical distinction to make is whether the DCIS is of the comedo- or noncomedo type.

Table 3-3. Differential features of carcinoma in situ

	Comedo-type DCIS	Noncomedo-type DCIS	Lobular carcinoma in situ
Mammographic features	Coarsely granular and casting calcifications	Finely granular calcifications	None
Tumor size >5 cm	Frequent	Few	Few
Presence of necrosis	Frequent	Occasional	Uncommon
Cell size	Large	Moderate	Small
Nuclear features	Pleomorphic, high grade	Minimal pleomorphism	Uniform, round
Prognosis	Worse than other types	Average	Bilateral cancer risk

DCIS = ductal carcinoma in situ.

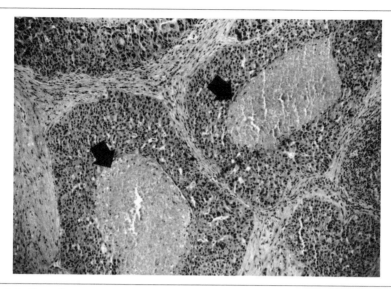

Fig. 3-6. Comedo-type ductal carcinoma in situ. Note the central necrosis marked by arrows (H&E, 250×).

Comedo-type DCIS (comedocarcinoma) (Fig. 3-6) acquired its name because it grossly resembles a comedone. These lesions are characterized microscopically by distended ducts and lobules, large cells, and high-grade pleomorphic nuclei. The center of the distended ducts and lobules are filled with abundant necrotic debris that can appear grossly cheesy (thus the name "comedo"). This necrotic debris calcifies, appearing mammographically as coarsely granular or "casting" calcifications because they outline the involved duct. Ninety-four percent of all comedocarcinomas will be evident on mammogram. However, mammography typically underestimates their size. A large percentage of comedo-type lesions are 5 cm or more. It is therefore important that these lesions be widely excised and that the surgical margins are carefully examined microscopically by the pathologist for the presence of tumor. Involvement of a surgical margin by tumor may preclude breast conserving treatment (see Chap. 13). Microinvasion is also common in these large lesions, and 1% to 2% will have axillary metastases, even if invasion is not demonstrable with extensive microscopic sampling.

Comedo-type DCIS is associated with a poorer prognosis than non-comedo-type DCIS. This correlates with other poor prognostic features such as high-grade nuclei and the fact that many of these lesions are positive for the oncoprotein Her-2-Neu.

Noncomedo-type DCIS includes lesions classified as micropapillary (Fig. 3-7), cribriform (Fig. 3-5B), solid, or clinging. They are characterized by the following: (1) solid distention of the involved ducts and lobules by smaller, uniform, monotonous cells that do not have the high-grade nuclei; (2) lack of central necrosis; and (3) the presence of rigid geometric spaces and bridges within the involved

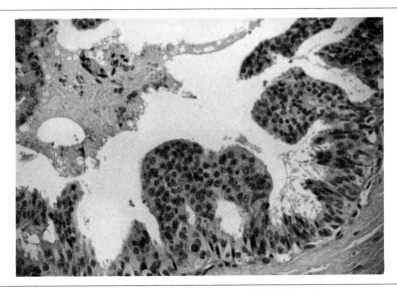

Fig. 3-7. Micropapillary ductal carcinoma in situ (H&E, 250×).

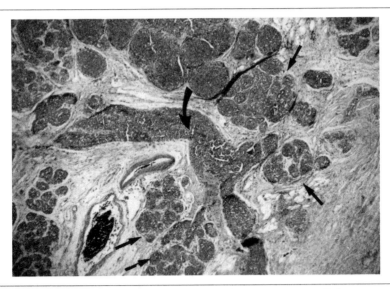

Fig. 3-8. Lobular carcinoma in situ is characterized by a solid cellular proliferation in the lobules *(small arrows)* with extension into the ducts *(curved arrow)* (H&E, 100×).

ducts and lobules. Noncomedo-type DCIS also frequently presents on mammography as microcalcifications (though less frequently than comedo-type) and fine granular calcifications rather than the coarsely granular, casting type of calcification are apparent.

LOBULAR CARCINOMA IN SITU. Lobular carcinoma in situ (LCIS) (Fig. 3-8) is usually an incidental finding in breast tissue removed for another indication and is frequently multifocal. This lesion rarely causes changes in the physical exam or mammographic abnormalities, but is a histologic marker of increased breast cancer risk in either breast. It is characterized microscopically by distention of at least half of the acini in a lobular unit by a population of round, uniform, small cells that may have clear cytoplasm or nuclear vacuoles. Similar-appearing cells may also be noted immediately above the basement membrane in larger ducts, displacing the normal ductal cells, which are pushed up. This is referred to as *pagetoid involvement of the ducts.*

Major Types of Breast Carcinoma and Their Clinical Significance

Infiltrating ductal carcinoma (Fig. 3-9) is the most common type of invasive breast cancer, accounting for 50% to 75% of cases, and is sometimes referred to as "carcinoma of no special type." There are many histologic and cytologic patterns within this category, and grading these features can help determine prognosis (see Chap. 5). In general, this category has a worse prognosis than those of special type (i.e., mucinous, tubular, or papillary carcinomas) (Table 3-4).

 Mucinous, tubular, and papillary carcinomas are all special types of ductal carcinoma considered to be well-differentiated subtypes that have an improved rate of survival. *Mucinous (colloid) carcinoma* (Fig. 3-10) accounts for 2% of all breast cancers, is rare in women under age 35, and is characterized by the production of abundant pools of mucin that make this tumor feel deceptively soft and benign.

Fig. 3-9. Infiltrating ductal carcinoma (H&E, 250×).

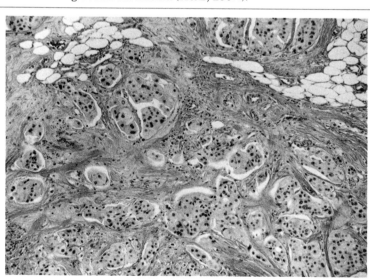

Table 3-4. Features of common breast carcinomas

	Type of carcinoma					
	Ductal (no special type)	Mucinous	Tubular	Papillary	Medullary	Lobular
Nuclear atypia	Variable	Minimal	Minimal	Variable	Marked	Minimal
Characteristic histology	None	Mucin production	Formation of tubules	Frondlike structure	Syncytia, lymphoid infiltration	Single-file arrangement
Clinical features	Hard	Soft, well circumscribed	Small	Soft, cystic	Soft, well circumscribed	Hard
Prognosis	Variable	Good	Best	Good	Good	Intermediate

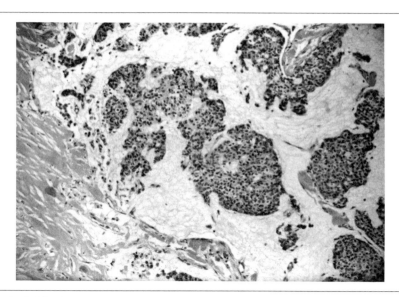

Fig. 3-10. Mucinous carcinoma. Note the well-differentiated nests of tumor floating in pools of mucin (H&E, 250×).

It is usually well circumscribed, and the tumor cells show little atypia. *Tubular carcinoma* is the most well-differentiated form of breast cancer, frequently presents as small, occult lesions discovered by screening mammography, and is usually curable. Tubular carcinoma derives its name from well-defined oval or round tubular structures formed by cells with little atypia. Because this lesion is so well differentiated, it can be difficult to distinguish microscopically from sclerosing adenosis and other benign sclerosing lesions. *Papillary carcinoma* (Fig. 3-11) usually occurs in large ducts and shares the frondlike branching structure of the benign papilloma. Unlike the benign papilloma, however, papillary carcinoma is lined by closely packed stratified cells with nuclear atypia. This cancer may occur in a cyst and can be either in situ or associated with well-differentiated invasive components.

Medullary carcinoma (Fig. 3-12) is another subtype of ductal carcinoma associated with a better-than-average prognosis. It is characterized histologically by syncytial sheets of large pleomorphic cells with a prominent lymphoid infiltrate. These tumors are usually well circumscribed with little fibrous reaction; thus, medullary carcinoma can also feel deceptively soft and benign. Necrosis is common, but does not usually calcify.

Infiltrating lobular carcinoma (Fig. 3-13) is characterized histologically by small cells, which frequently contain a cytoplasmic vacuole and are classically arranged in a single-file ("Indian-file") arrangement. The stroma is densely sclerotic giving this tumor a rock-hard feeling on palpation and making the cells difficult to remove by fine needle aspiration. This tumor has an intermediate

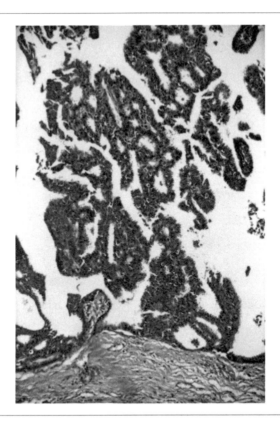

Fig. 3-11. Frondlike configuration characteristic of papillary carcinoma (H&E, 100×).

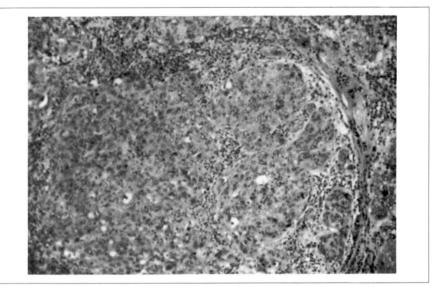

Fig. 3-12. Medullary carcinoma. Note the sheetlike arrangement of the cells and lymphocytic infiltrate (H&E, 100×).

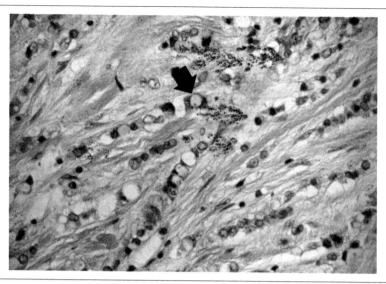

Fig. 3-13. Infiltrating lobular carcinoma. Unlike the ductal carcinoma shown in Fig. 3-9, this carcinoma is characterized by smaller cell size and linear arrangement of cells. Many cells have a cytoplasmic vacuole containing mucin *(arrow),* characteristic of this tumor type (H&E, 250×).

prognosis in its classic form (variants do exist) and has an increased incidence of multifocality and bilaterality.

Rare forms of breast carcinoma include tumors that resemble salivary gland cancers, such as adenoid cystic carcinoma, which has an excellent prognosis, and mucoepidermoid carcinoma, whose prognosis is similar to ductal carcinomas of no special type. Secretory carcinoma contains intercellular and extracellular secretions and has an excellent prognosis in young women. Metaplastic carcinomas have a poor prognosis, are characterized by sarcomatous differentiation of the malignant epithelium, and may include osteosarcomatous, chondrosarcomatous, and fibrosarcomatous elements.

Stromal Tumors of the Breast

Stromal tumors, and in particular sarcomas, are considerably less common than epithelial lesions of the breast. These should be distinguished from carcinomas with sarcomatoid metaplasia because patient management is different. Sarcomas of the breast are rare and include, among others, angiosarcoma, leiomyosarcoma, and malignant fibrous histiocytoma. The most common stromal tumor is the phyllodes tumor.

Phyllodes Tumors

The term *phyllodes tumor* replaced the former misleading term *cystosarcoma phyllodes* when it was recognized that this tumor has a spectrum of histopathologic appearances and biologic behaviors ranging from benign to malignant. While often large, these tumors may be as small as 1 to 2 cm, and may have a cystic component. Phyllodes tumors are rare in adolescents; they usually occur in women in the fifth decade of life, older than those in whom fibroadenomas are usually seen. They have been diagnosed in women as old as 70.

Microscopically, phyllodes tumors resemble fibroadenomas in that they both represent a proliferation of stromal and glandular elements. The phyllodes tumor, however, can be distinguished from fibroadenoma by a hypercellular stroma that often shows a cambium layer near the epithelium. Malignant phyllodes tumors are characterized by the presence of a stroma that resembles a sarcomatous stroma, and by the presence of more than 10 mitoses per high power field. The stroma may resemble a fibrosarcoma or have heterologous elements such as malignant bone or cartilage, rhabdomyosarcoma, or liposarcoma. The borders may be infiltrating or circumscribed. Malignant phyllodes tumors metastasize hematogenously, are locally invasive, and spread along nerves. A tumor with a sarcomatous stroma, but with only 5 to 9 mitoses per high power field denotes a phyllodes tumor of borderline malignant potential. Most borderline tumors are cured by excision, but they may recur or metastasize. Transformation to a frankly malignant tumor occurs in only 7% of cases.

Suggested Reading

General

Breast cancer research: A special report. *Science* 259:616–638, 1993.

Diet

Goodwin PJ, and Boyd NF. Critical appraisal of the evidence that dietary fat intake is related to breast cancer risk in humans. *J Natl Cancer Inst* 79:473–485, 1987.

Howe GR, et al. Dietary factors and risk of breast cancer: Combined analysis of 12 case-controlled studies. *J Natl Cancer Inst* 82:561–569, 1990.

Jones D, et al. Dietary fat and breast cancer in the National Health and Nutrition Examination Survey I. Epidemiological Follow-up Study. *J Natl Cancer Inst* 79:465–471, 1987.

Kritchevsky D. Nutrition and breast cancer. *Cancer* 66:1321–1325, 1990.

Genetics

King MC. Linkage of early-onset familial breast cancer to chromosome 17q21. *Science* 250:1684, 1990.

King MC. Breast cancer genes: How many, where, and who are they? *Nature Genetics* 2:125, 1992.

Rosen PP, et al. Epidemiology of breast carcinoma III: Relationship of family history to tumor type. *Cancer* 50:171–179, 1982.

Sattin RW, et al. Family history and the risk of breast cancer. *JAMA* 253:1908–1913, 1985.

Breast Pathology

Consensus Meeting, Cancer Committee of the College of American Pathologists. Is "fibrocystic disease" of the breast precancerous? *Arch Pathol Lab Med* 110:171–172, 1986.

London SJ, et al. A prospective study of benign breast disease and the risk of breast cancer. *JAMA* 267:941–944, 1992.

Page DL, and Anderson TJ. *Diagnostic Histopathology of the Breast.* New York: Churchill Livingstone, 1987.

Pietruszka M, and Barnes L. Cystosarcoma phyllodes: A clinico-pathologic analysis of 42 cases. *Cancer* 41:1974–1983, 1978.

Rosai J. Borderline epithelial lesions of the breast. *Am J Surg Pathol* 15:209–221, 1991.

Schnitt S, et al. Interobserver reproducibility in the diagnosis of ductal proliferative breast lesions using standardized criteria. *Am J Surg Pathol* 16:1133–1143, 1992.

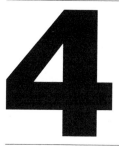

Screening for Breast Cancer

Karen K. Lindfors

Mammography

Increased emphasis has been placed on breast cancer screening over the last several years. The media have focused much attention, both positive and negative, on mammography in particular. Women have become better educated about the advantages of mammography and efforts have been made to reduce the cost and improve quality, yet compliance with established screening guidelines, even in women over age 50, is poor. While nearly 75% of women over age 40 have had at least one mammogram, less than one-third receive screening at regular intervals. Fear of cancer and discomfort as well as the cost and inconvenience of mammography can be deterrents, but the reason most frequently cited by women who do not receive routine mammographic screening is that their primary physician does not recommend it. The National Cancer Institute's year 2000 goal is 80% participation in regular mammographic screening for breast cancer. Physician education is the key to reaching this goal.

Survival from breast cancer is influenced by tumor size, degree of invasion, and lymph node status at the time of diagnosis. It is well known that mammography can image very small cancers frequently before they invade surrounding tissues or metastasize to lymph nodes. In many cases, the cancers seen mammographically are not palpable, even when their location is provided by the mammogram. It can be anticipated, therefore, that a regular program of mammographic screening should lower mortality from breast cancer. Other benefits of mammographic screening include the ability to perform breast conserving therapy in women with small tumors and a reduced need for systemic therapy in such women.

Although mammography is an excellent tool for the detection of breast cancer, not all cancers can be imaged mammographically. In young patients with dense breasts the false-negative rate of mammography may approach 25%. In older women with fatty replaced breasts the false-negative rate is much lower, about 5% to 6%. Because mammography is imperfect and is not routinely used in all women, breast physical examination by physicians and breast self-examination by the patient must also remain an integral part of any breast cancer screening program.

Clinical Trials and Efficacy Studies

Health Insurance Plan of New York

In 1963 the Health Insurance Plan of New York (HIP) invited 31,000 women aged 40 to 64 to participate in four annual screenings for breast cancer by mammography and physical examination. The group undergoing screening was compared with a control group who received routine medical care. Nine years after beginning the study there was a 29% reduction in breast cancer mortality in the group receiving annual screening (Table 4-1).

European Studies

Several other breast cancer screening trials were begun in Europe in the 1970s. In Sweden, the Two County Study was a randomized population-based trial of screening for breast cancer with single-view mammography alone. The screening intervals ranged from 24 to 33 months. Eight years after the initiation of the program, breast cancer mortality in the screened group was reduced by 31%.

Not all clinical trials have shown significant reductions in breast cancer mortality with mammographic screening. In Malmö, Sweden, a population-based randomized trial was performed that included 42,000 women from ages 45 to 79. After 9 years no significant difference between the study and control groups was evident, yet when screened women over age 55 were examined separately they had a 20% reduction in breast cancer mortality. It is difficult to understand the difference in results between the Malmö and the Two County studies. Hypotheses for the varying results include a higher rate of

Table 4-1. Randomized clinical trials of breast cancer screening (5- to 13-year follow-up)

Trial	Breast cancer mortality reduction in those screened	Type of screening
HIP	29%	Annual two-view mammogram + BPE
Swedish Two County	31%	Single view mammogram every 2–3 years
Malmö	0	Initial two-view mammogram, then single- or two-view mammogram every 18–24 months
Canadian NBSS	0	Annual two-view mammogram + BPE
Combined Swedish Trials	24%	Mammogram at variable intervals

HIP = Health Insurance Plan (of New York); BPE = breast physical examination; NBSS = National Breast Screening Study.

mammography among the controls in Malmö and a lower compliance with screening among the study population in that trial.

A 1993 follow-up study was based on pooled data from all of the Swedish randomized screening trials. This overview, based on a 5- to 13-year follow-up of nearly 283,000 women in five geographic areas of the country, demonstrated a statistically significant 24% reduction in mortality from breast cancer among women invited to mammographic screening.

Several case-controlled studies have added evidence in support of mammographic screening as a way to reduce mortality from breast cancer. Two such studies were performed in the Netherlands and one was done in Italy. In all three, women who died from breast cancer were matched to women who did not die from the disease and the use of screening mammography was studied. The relative risk of dying from breast cancer in screened women versus unscreened women ranged from .30 to .53. These results suggest that mammographic screening can reduce breast cancer deaths by 47% to 70%.

Canadian National Breast Screening Study

Although the majority of data support screening mammography, the Canadian National Breast Screening Study (NBSS), a randomized clinical trial performed in almost 90,000 women ages 40 to 59 and published in late 1992, was not able to demonstrate a reduction in mortality from breast cancer among women undergoing mammography. The NBSS differed from other trials in that the control group for women over 50 received annual breast physical examination. Results were published after 7 years of follow-up.

Even before the NBSS was published, serious questions were raised about the validity of its results. To be effective, mammography must be performed in a technically optimal manner and results must be interpreted by a radiologist with expertise in this area. Half of the mammograms performed during the first 2 years of the Canadian study were judged technically unacceptable by an outside panel of reviewers. Breast positioning and image quality were among the criteria reviewed. Additionally, an external review of over 5000 mammograms from the study demonstrated a high number of false-negative interpretations by study radiologists. Thirty-five percent of all interval cancers and 17% of all screening detected cancers were false-negatives at the previous screening. There were further criticisms about the randomization process and short follow-up time.

Age Recommendations

Most organizations recommend annual mammography and clinical breast examination in women aged 50 and over (Table 4-2). There is still controversy over the benefit of screening mammography in women in their forties because stratification of trial results by age shows limited evidence to support screening in this age group.

Table 4-2. Breast cancer screening guidelines*

Age (years)	Breast physical examination	Mammography
Beginning by age 40	Annual	Every 1–2 years
50 and over	Annual	Annual

*Endorsed by the following:
  American Association of Women Radiologists
  American Cancer Society
  American College of Radiology
  American Medical Association
  American Osteopathic College of Radiology
  American Society for Therapeutic Radiology and Oncology
  American Society of Clinical Oncology
  American Society of Internal Medicine
  College of American Pathologists
  National Medical Association

The American College of Obstetricians and Gynecologists endorses these guidelines, but also recommends a baseline mammogram between the ages of 35 and 40.

Women in Their Forties

RESEARCH RESULTS. The debate regarding the benefit of mammographic screening for women 40 to 49 years of age intensified after publication of the Canadian NBSS in late 1992. In this trial, which has been the only one specifically designed to examine this age group, no significant reduction in breast cancer mortality occurred among those women who received annual mammography and breast physical examination when compared with unscreened women (Table 4-3). As discussed above, however, the results of the trial are marred by the serious criticisms leveled at its design and conduct.

The issue of whether to perform breast cancer screening in women between the ages of 40 and 49 is a difficult one. Unfortunately, all of the clinical trials have been flawed with respect to their ability to demonstrate a reduction in breast cancer mortality among screened women in this age group; inadequate follow-up time, small numbers of women in the appropriate age group, poor quality mammography, and faulty randomization have all been cited as reasons for the lack of absolute proof of a benefit from mammography. For the same reasons, however, there is no absolute proof of the converse, that no benefit results from mammographic screening in the 40- to 49-year-old age group.

When data randomized from clinical trials are stratified by age, and women age 40 to 49 are examined separately, the only significant mortality reduction due to screening mammography occurred at 18 years of follow-up in the HIP study. Screening women in this age group began to show a lower mortality from breast cancer after 10 to 12 years of follow-up. Until this point, there was no difference in mortality rates between screened and unscreened women.

The combined data from the Swedish screening trials show that

Table 4-3. Breast cancer mortality reductions, by age group

Trial (randomized, clinical)	Maximum follow-up period (years)	Mortality reduction	
		Younger (specific ages in years)	Older (specific ages in years)
HIP	18	24% (40–49)	21% (50–64)
Swedish Two County	7	0 (40–49)	39% (50–74)
Malmö	8	0 (45–55)	20% (55–79)
Canadian NBSS	7	0 (40–49)	0 (50–59)
Combined Swedish	13	13% (40–49)	29% (50–69)

HIP = Health Insurance Plan (of New York); NBSS = National Breast Screening Study.

for women age 40 to 49, there was a 13% decrease in mortality from breast cancer after 5 to 13 years of follow-up. This is not a statistically significant result, but it does roughly parallel what was seen in the HIP trial. None of the individual Swedish trials have been able to prove a conclusive benefit from screening in this age group.

Additional suggestive evidence of benefit for 40- to 49-year-old women from screening mammography was accrued by the Breast Cancer Detection Demonstration Project (BCDDP). In this noncontrolled study of volunteer women, one-third of breast cancers diagnosed occurred in women age 35 to 49. The majority of these cancers were noninvasive or did not involve regional lymph nodes; most were detected by mammography rather than by physical examination.

COST-BENEFIT ANALYSIS. Given that mammography has proved effective in women aged 50 and older, that there are trends that suggest probable benefit in women aged 40 to 49, and that it is not a harmful procedure (see section on Radiation Risk), the main deterrents to the performance of screening mammography in women aged 40 to 49 years are cost and the risk of a false-positive result. Can we afford to screen these younger women in whom the risk of contracting breast cancer is small? This is the real question that must be answered. The probability that a woman will develop breast cancer between ages 40 and 50 is about 13 in 1000; the probability of dying from the disease within 10 years for this age group is about 8 in 1000. This can be reduced to about 5 or 6 per 1000 if mammography is performed annually. The cost per year of life saved by screening in women aged 40 to 49 has been estimated at $27,000 if a breast cancer mortality reduction of 30% can be achieved through screening. The cost increases to about $140,000 with a 10% breast cancer mortality reduction.

RECOMMENDATIONS. The American College of Physicians (ACP) recommends annual screening for breast cancer with breast physical examination and mammography for all asymptomatic women over age 50. Mammography is not suggested for women between ages 40 and 49 unless they are at increased risk; however, annual breast physical examination is recommended for these women. The rationale for these recommendations is based on the conflicting evidence of the effectiveness of screening mammography in the younger group, the low incidence of cancer in women under 50, and the cost of screening. The ACP does, however, recommend counseling each woman on the benefits, risks, and costs of screening mammography so that she can choose the screening strategy that best suits her.

In late 1993, the National Cancer Institute withdrew its support for screening mammography in women under age 50. It cited a lack of proof of benefit from screening in this age group as the rationale for this decision. Revised guidelines for this age group have not been issued by the agency.

The American Cancer Society, as well as 10 other medical organizations (see Table 4-2), continue to recommend that screening mammography be performed every 1 to 2 years in 40- to 49-year-old women. The variable interval for this age group is, again, based mainly on economic grounds. Some experts believe that breast cancer is, however, more aggressive in younger women and that these women should be screened annually. Others suggest that women between the ages of 40 and 49 who are at high risk be screened annually, while those without such risk factors receive biennial mammograms. A close family history of breast cancer, a personal history of the disease, or previous breast biopsies showing atypical hyperplasia or lobular neoplasia are some of the factors that increase a woman's risk of contracting breast cancer.

Women Under Forty

In general, asymptomatic women under the age of 40 should not undergo routine screening mammography. There will be exceptions to this policy, especially when women have significant family histories of breast cancer (i.e., two or more first-degree relatives with the disease) or other significant risk factors (history of breast cancer, atypical hyperplasia, lobular neoplasia). In such cases, screening may begin during the fourth decade.

RECOMMENDATIONS. The American College of Obstetricians and Gynecologists continues to recommend one baseline mammogram between ages 35 and 40. Most other organizations have eliminated this recommendation. Radiologists generally feel that if regular screening mammography begins at age 40, a baseline study before this age is not essential. Judicious use of mammographic screening in women under age 35 to 40 is suggested by data showing increased susceptibility to breast cancer among women exposed to very high doses of radiation in their teens and twenties. These data combined with the low incidence of breast cancer in such women suggest that restricted use of screening mammography in women under age 35 to 40 is prudent.

At What Age Should Mammographic Screening Stop?

Most guidelines for breast cancer screening are open-ended; no specific age at which screening should be discontinued is recommended. Breast cancer incidence rises with age. Mammography is at least as effective in detecting early stage cancers in older women as it is in younger women. In fact, positive biopsy rates for mammographic findings in women over age 70 are nearly double the rates for women under age 50. Breast cancer appears to be as aggressive in the elderly as it is in other women, but there is no direct evidence showing a reduction in mortality from breast cancer through screening in women over age 75. Some studies have shown a decrease in mortality in women up to age 74; older women have not been studied.

So how does the clinician decide when screening should stop? Certainly, the life expectancy and quality of life of the patient must be taken into account. The clinician must assess the impact of comorbid conditions on the woman's ability to survive long enough to benefit from breast cancer screening. It may make sense to screen a relatively healthy 75-year-old who still has a life expectancy of 12 years, while it may not be reasonable to screen a woman the same age with severe cardiac disease.

Once the clinician has decided to screen the patient, the frequency of such screening must be determined. Studies have shown effectiveness of intervals ranging from 12 to 33 months. The federal government has made the decision for some women because current policy provides Medicare reimbursement only for biennial mammographic screening in women aged 65 and over. The American Cancer Society, however, still recommends annual screening in women of these ages provided that their general health is good.

Recommendations

A recent forum convened to study breast cancer screening in older women made the following recommendations: (1) for women 65 through 74 years of age, clinical breast examination should be performed every year, and mammography should be performed approximately every two years, and (2) for women 75 years and older, whose general health and life expectancy are good, similar recommendations are made. Unfortunately, there is no simple answer to the question, "At what age should screening be stopped?" Clinicians will have to weigh each case individually.

Radiation Risk

No documented radiation-induced breast cancer from mammographic screening has ever been reported. There is, however, evidence to suggest that among women exposed to high doses of radiation (100–2000 cGy or rads) there is an excess risk of breast cancer.

Survivors of the atomic bombs in Japan, patients undergoing radiation therapy for benign breast conditions in New York and Sweden, and tuberculosis victims who underwent multiple chest fluoroscopies for monitoring of therapeutic response in Canada and Massachusetts are three populations in whom an increased incidence of breast cancer have been documented. These data raise questions about the impact of the radiation received during mammographic screening on the incidence of breast cancer.

Estimating the risk of breast cancer from the low doses of radiation received during mammography is complex. On the average, the mean glandular dose to each breast is 2.5 mGy (.25 rad) when a two-view mammographic study is performed. A controlled study to determine the effect of such low doses of radiation on the incidence of breast cancer would require huge numbers of women in both exposed and nonexposed groups. Over 10 million women in each group would be required to offer enough statistical power for analysis. Clearly, such a study would be impossible. As a result, current estimates of radiation risk from mammography are based on extrapolation from higher doses. The most recent hypothetical risks were calculated in 1990 by the National Research Council Committee on the Biological Effects of Ionizing Radiation (BEIR V). The report from this committee concluded that there is little evidence of any increased risk to women exposed after age 40.

Using a linear dose-response model and pooling data from the atomic bomb survivors and the Massachusetts fluoroscopy and New York radiotherapy incidence series, BEIR V developed a time-dependent relative-risk model for both breast cancer incidence and mortality. Data presented in this report show that mammographic examination of 1 million women at age 45 would theoretically result in five excess breast cancer deaths among those women during their lifetimes (Table 4-4). This risk of death is equal to that incurred by one coast-to-coast round-trip airline trip, a 450-mile car trip, or smoking three cigarettes. As women age, there is a progressive reduction in this hypothetical risk of death from radiation-induced cancers.

Risk Versus Potential Benefits

To further place the hypothetical risks of mammography into context, they must be weighed against the potential benefits of screening (Table 4-5). In a group of 1 million 45-year-old women, about 750 deaths from breast cancer are expected. Assuming a 20% reduction in mortality from screening mammography, 150 deaths could be averted by screening. If a 40% reduction in mortality by screening is assumed, 300 deaths could be averted. Clearly, the benefits gained by screening are far greater than the theoretical risks. As women age, the benefits become even greater because there is an increased

Table 4-4. Hypothetical risk of death from breast cancer due to radiogenic and nonradiogenic tumors in women age 45

Cause of death	Deaths per million women
Radiogenic breast cancer induced by mammography	5
Nonradiogenic breast cancer among women undergoing mammography (assuming a 20% mortality reduction due to screening)	600
Nonradiogenic breast cancer among unscreened women	750

incidence of breast cancer and a reduced hypothetical risk from mammography. Subsequent annual screening can also reduce the hypothetical risk of dying from a radiogenic breast cancer because some of these cancers will be detected at an earlier, more curable stage.

Physical Examination and Breast Self-Examination

For patients over the age of 40 with no particular risk of breast disease, a thorough physical examination of the breasts should be done yearly. For women at high risk of developing breast cancer (i.e., history of breast cancer, atypical hyperplasia, lobular neoplasia) this interval should be shortened to 4 months. Clinical examination and mammography are complementary. Both are necessary for maximum effectiveness of a screening program.

No matter how skilled or caring the physician, it is impossible to remember every area of nodularity in the breast of every patient. Comparison of sequential clinical breast examination can, therefore, be difficult. There are no randomized trials demonstrating the efficacy of breast self-examination (BSE), but experience shows it can be helpful. If the patient is trained adequately in BSE, she can become familiar with her own unique "lumps and bumps" and can call attention to changes. Many studies have shown that the most effective teacher of BSE is the physician, if she or he teaches the patient as part of the yearly examination and reinforces the teaching periodically. The second most effective teacher is another health professional, and the third most effective (but still excellent) are the trained volunteers of American Cancer Society units.

There are several breast self-examination techniques, all acceptable. Video tapes and brochures are available from your local unit of the American Cancer Society (see Appendix A). Lifelike plastic models containing palpable lesions are available from medical supply houses and are effective teaching tools.

Table 4-5. Hypothetical deaths averted by mammographic screening in women age 45

Breast cancer mortality reduction due to screening	Deaths averted per million women
20%	150
40%	300

The Use of Other Imaging Modalities for Screening

Mammography is the only imaging modality with proven capability to screen asymptomatic women for breast cancer. *Ultrasound* was investigated as a possible alternative, but did not prove effective. Less than half of all breast cancers can be visualized sonographically. Ultrasound is useful only to further characterize a specific lesion detected by mammography or physical examination. Its main utility lies in distinguishing simple cysts from solid or complex masses. Ultrasound cannot replace mammography in breast cancer screening.

Thermography and *transillumination* are two other imaging techniques that have been studied for potential use as screening modalities. Neither has proved useful for the detection or diagnosis of breast cancer.

Recent interest has been focused on *magnetic resonance imaging* (MRI) as a possible alternative to mammography. Preliminary data suggest that MRI with contrast can reveal lesions in dense breasts that may be missed by conventional mammograms. The cost of MRI and the time required to perform it will likely prohibit its use for general screening, but it may prove to be a useful ancillary technique to mammography.

Technical and Quality Assurance Aspects of Mammographic Screening

Effective breast cancer screening in asymptomatic women depends on high-quality mammography and thorough clinical breast examination. Mammography must be performed on a dedicated unit, that is, an x-ray unit specifically designed for this purpose. Mammography units have x-ray tubes to generate the low-energy photons that are necessary for high-contrast images. In this way tissues that are inherently similar in density (i.e., fat, ductal tissue, masses, etc.) can be discriminated. Dedicated mammography units are designed to produce images with high spatial resolution so that tiny microcalcifications can be seen.

All mammographic units are equipped with compression paddles that squeeze the breast against the film holders. Such compression is applied for only a few seconds while the film is exposed. Firm compression of the breast is essential for the production of high-quality films. It prevents blurring from patient motion, and it spreads overlapping tissues apart so that abnormalities can be seen more clearly. Compression also creates a more uniform thickness of the breast so that the film will be properly exposed in all areas. The amount of radiation received by the patient can also be reduced by good compression; a thinner breast requires fewer x-ray photons to create an image.

Women need to be informed about the necessity and advantages of compression during mammography. Those who are prepared for the examination seem to have less discomfort. Reassurance that mammography is not painful can reduce the chance that pain will be perceived during the procedure. It is important that referring physicians discuss this issue with their patients, so that women will not hesitate to follow recommendations for mammography.

Other factors necessary to ensure a high-quality mammographic screening program include the type of film and screens used, the film processing system, the expertise of the technologist, and the experience and knowledge of the interpreting radiologist.

The American College of Radiology (ACR) has established national quality assurance standards for mammography through its Mammography Accreditation Program. Accreditation of a mammography facility by the ACR is currently the best assurance a woman and her physician can have that a high-quality examination and interpretation will result when a women undergoes mammography. Other specific quality assurance programs have been implemented by some states. Up to this time ACR accreditation has been voluntary, but the recent passage of the federal Mammography Quality Standards Act has mandated accreditation of all facilities by October 1994. Federal standards for accreditation will probably be similar to those of the ACR program.

The Screening Mammogram

The screening mammogram usually consists of two views of each breast: the mediolateral oblique (MLO) and the craniocaudal (CC) views.

Mediolateral Oblique View

The *MLO view,* when properly performed, depicts the most breast tissue; it is orientated parallel to the patient's pectoralis major muscle (Fig. 4-1). The angle of obliquity can vary, but is generally between 40 and 60 degrees. The technologist is given flexibility in

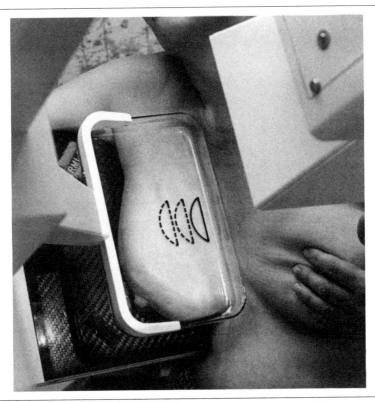

Fig. 4-1. A patient who has been positioned for a mediolateral oblique mammogram. The film cassette and the compression paddle are oriented parallel to the pectoralis major muscle.

choosing the angle so that the greatest amount of breast tissue can be visualized.

A properly positioned MLO view should show the pectoralis major muscle down to the level of the nipple. The inframammary fold should be visualized to ensure that inferior tissues have been adequately imaged. The nipple should be in profile so that the subareolar area can be evaluated (Fig. 4-2). By standard convention, markers indicating the side (left or right) and the type of view (MLO) should be placed near the superior axillary tissues of the breast. In some practices the MLO view may be marked as an oblique or axillary view.

Craniocaudal View

The *CC view* images the breast in the superior to inferior direction (Fig. 4-3). Sometimes the curvature of the chest wall hinders imaging of some of the lateral or medial tissue in the CC projection. When evaluating a CC view, optimal positioning can be best ensured by

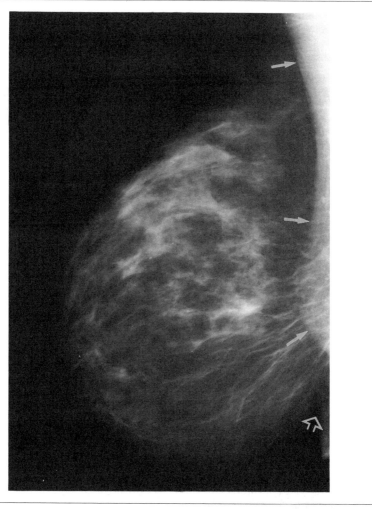

Fig. 4-2. A properly positioned right mediolateral oblique (MLO) mammogram. The pectoralis muscle *(straight arrows)* can be followed to the level of the nipple and the inframammary fold *(open arrow)* is also seen. The nipple is in profile and can only be seen if a bright light is used to illuminate the skin.

sighting the pectoralis muscles at the edge of the film (Fig. 4-4); unfortunately, this is not always possible due to differences in body habitus among patients. One must rely on the expertise of the technologist to ensure that the maximum amount of tissue has been visualized. The depth of tissue seen on the CC view should be similar to the depth of tissue seen anterior to the pectoralis on the MLO view. In the CC view, as in the MLO view, the nipple should be in profile. Markers indicating the side (left or right) and view (CC) are placed adjacent to the lateral tissues. Proper marker placement is the only

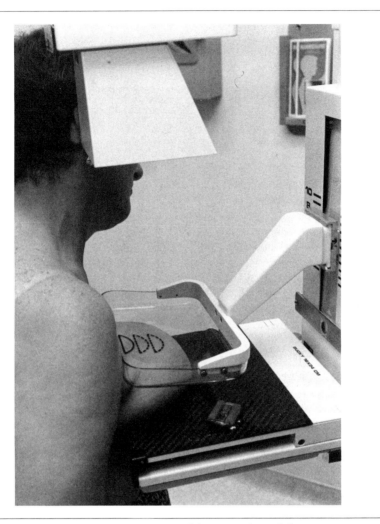

Fig. 4-3. A patient who has been positioned for a craniocaudal mammogram. The film is located under the breast and the compression paddle is applied to the superior skin surface.

sure method of determining what is lateral and what is medial on a CC view.

Additional Views

Other mammographic views may be required to clarify potential areas of abnormality (see Chap. 6). Occasionally these will be performed immediately after the screening mammogram. More frequently, in the interests of keeping costs low, all screening mammograms are read by the radiologist once or twice a day in batches; thus, if clarification is needed the woman will have to return to the radiology office on another day for additional views.

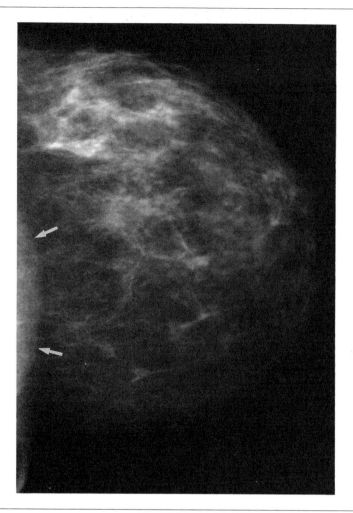

Fig. 4-4. A properly positioned left craniocaudal (CC) mammogram. The pectoralis muscle *(arrows)* is visualized along the chest wall. The nipple is in profile and can only be seen when a bright light is used to illuminate the skin.

Outcomes

There are three basic outcomes in screening mammography: (1) a negative study in which there is no mammographic evidence of cancer, (2) a positive study for which further tests (i.e., additional views, ultrasound, or biopsy) are recommended, and (3) a screening examination showing an area that is highly likely to be benign, but for which a short interval follow-up mammogram is recommended. (See Chap. 6 for discussion of positive screening studies and those for which short interval follow-up is recommended.)

A *negative screening mammogram* is just one component of a negative screen for breast cancer. Mammography has a false-negative

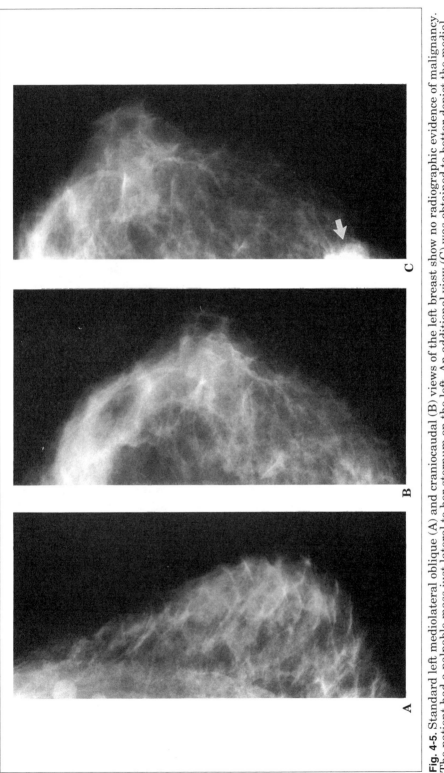

Fig. 4-5. Standard left mediolateral oblique (A) and craniocaudal (B) views of the left breast show no radiographic evidence of malignancy. The patient had a palpable mass just lateral to her sternum on the left. An additional view (C) was obtained to better depict the medial tissues close to the chest wall. An infiltrating duct carcinoma *(arrow)*, which had not been seen on standard screening views, is partially visualized. (Courtesy of Dr. Denny Anspach, Sacramento, California.)

rate of 8% to 10%, so effective screening must also include a high-quality physical examination of the breasts. Clinicians must be cautioned not to ignore a suspicious palpable abnormality, even if the mammogram is negative.

False-negative mammograms can occur for a variety of reasons. The palpable abnormality may not be included in the area of the breast that is filmed: Masses that are close to the chest wall can be difficult to image (Fig. 4-5). The particular tumor type may not be visible mammographically. The filming technique may be suboptimal or there may be observer error in the interpretation of the mammogram. Dense breast parenchyma may obscure visualization of a mass; physical examination is particularly important when the radiologist reports that the patient's breasts are dense because the sensitivity of mammography may be even lower in these women. It must be emphasized that *a negative mammogram should not deter further diagnostic evaluation of a palpable mass.*

Women should be strongly advised that any palpable breast masses that occur in the interval between mammograms should be brought to the attention of their physician. The rate of interval cancers will depend on the frequency of screening. Interval cancers may be more biologically aggressive and tend to be more advanced at diagnosis than are cancers detected by screening.

About 10% of women undergoing screening mammography will have positive studies. Additional work-up will be recommended in these patients. The majority of these women will not require a biopsy after additional views or ultrasound (see Chap. 6 for further discussion).

Short-interval follow-up may be recommended after additional radiologic work-up has been performed. In some cases the radiologist may recommend such follow-up without any additional imaging. It is important that these women return for follow-up at the recommended schedule even though the likelihood of malignancy is 1% or less in such cases (see Chap. 6 for further discussion).

Suggested Reading

Andersson I, et al. Mammographic screening and mortality from breast cancer: the Malmö screening trial. *Br Med J* 297:943–948, 1988.

Baker, LH. Breast cancer detection demonstration project: Five year summary report. *Cancer* 32:194–225, 1982.

Chu, KC, Smart, CR, and Tarone, RE. Analysis of breast cancer mortality and stage distribution by age for the health insurance plan clinical trial. *J Natl Cancer Inst* 80:1125–1132, 1988.

Costanza, ME. Breast cancer screening in older women. Synopsis of a forum. *Cancer Suppl* 69:1925–1931, 1992.

Dodd, GD. American Cancer Society guidelines on screening for breast cancer. *Cancer Suppl* 69:1885–1887, 1992.

Feig, SA, and Hendrick, RE. Risk, Benefit, and Controversies in Mammographic Screening. In AG Haus and MJ Yaffe (eds), *Syllabus: A Categorical Course in Physics: Technical Aspects of Breast Imaging.* Oak Brook, IL: RSNA Publications, 1992, pp. 103–118.

Miller AB, et al. Canadian National Breast Screening Study. *Can Med Assoc J* 147:1459–1488, 1992.

Nyström L, et al. Breast cancer screening with mammography: Overview of Swedish randomised trials. *Lancet* 341:973–978, 1993.

Tabar L, et al. Reduction in mortality from breast cancer after mass screening with mammography: randomised trial from the Breast Cancer Screening Work Group of the Swedish National Board of Health and Welfare. *Lancet* i:829–832, 1985.

The Biopsy

Lydia Pleotis Howell

The majority of palpable breast lumps are not malignant, but it is often difficult to definitively make that determination by palpation or mammography or both. Many delays in breast cancer diagnosis occur because breast masses are followed clinically without microscopic evaluation. The best clinical plan for a patient with a breast mass is based on tissue diagnosis. While surgical excision is classically considered to be the gold standard, this is not always practical or desirable, due to cost, morbidity, and the frequent multifocal nature of breast masses requiring multiple surgical procedures. In this chapter, different biopsy methods for the evaluation of breast masses are discussed, including their advantages, disadvantages, and the tissue handling requirements that may be necessary for special prognostic studies. In addition, a special section addresses the surgical pathology report with the goal of helping the clinician glean all the information that the pathologist wishes to convey.

Biopsy Methods

Fine Needle Aspiration

Fine needle aspiration (FNA) biopsy is a simple technique. It should be performed after a mammogram because the hematoma it forms can interfere with mammographic interpretation. Equipment and technique for this procedure are listed in Tables 5-1 and 5-2 and illustrated in Figs. 5-1 and 5-2. In the United States, it is chiefly performed by primary care physicians and surgeons. However, it is becoming popular for pathologists to perform FNAs as is typical in Europe. FNA requires practice, and the best results are obtained by those who do it frequently. There are several important aspects to be considered in the performance of this procedure. Patients are very anxious when seeing a physician, especially for procedures involving a needle. The syringe and needle are best kept out of sight when possible. The syringe holder can look particularly intimidating, and it may be preferable to perform the aspiration without it, using instead a smaller 3-cc syringe that can be more easily concealed and manipulated with one hand. Because three to four passes are required to obtain an adequate sample, a local anesthetic (e.g., subcutaneous lidocaine injection) may be desired to minimize the pain with each needle stick. To obtain a representative sample, it is important to direct the needle into multiple areas within the mass when performing the aspiration (see Fig. 5-2).

The amount of material obtained during aspiration is very small and will be confined to the barrel of the needle. Do not expect to see any material in the syringe itself, unless cyst fluid is drained. If blood appears in the hub of the needle, stop aspirating and remove the needle and syringe to avoid further bloody contamination and potential hematoma formation. When withdrawing the needle, be sure to release negative pressure by letting go of the plunger. Otherwise, the sample will be contaminated by normal surrounding tissue as the needle is withdrawn from the mass, and air will be sucked into the syringe. The air will pull the scanty specimen into the barrel of the syringe where it is difficult, if not impossible, to expel.

The aspirated material should be expelled forcefully onto the glass slides, spread quickly into a thin layer, and fixed (Fig. 5-3). Be sure that the smear preparation and fixation occur as quickly as possible because poor preservation and air-drying artifacts can prevent adequate evaluation.

It is important to ascertain that the needle has penetrated the mass in question. Adequate stabilization of the mass, confidence in

Table 5-1. Equipment for fine needle aspiration biopsy

22-gauge needle attached to 3-cc syringe or 10-cc syringe in a syringe holder
Clear glass slides
Alcohol pads
Fixative if Papanicolaou stain is desired (95% ethanol or spray fixative)
Gauze pads
Adhesive bandage
Quick stain (e.g., toluidine blue O or Diff-Quik)
Coverslips

Table 5-2. How to perform fine needle aspiration biopsy

Cleanse site with ethanol
Stabilize mass between two fingers, if palpable
Insert needle into mass
Withdraw plunger to apply negative pressure
Direct needle into multiple areas within the mass
Release negative pressure
Withdraw needle
Remove needle
Pull back plunger
Reattach the needle
Expel material onto clean slides
Fix if desired
Stain with quick stain and examine microscopically
Repeat procedure 2 to 3 times

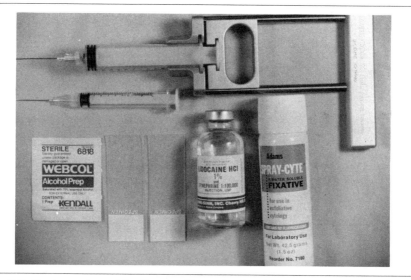

Fig. 5-1. Equipment used for fine needle aspiration. The pistol-grip needle holder at the top is used with a 10-cc syringe. Alternatively, a 3-cc syringe can be used alone.

needle placement, and resistance to the aspirating needle all are important to the diagnostic process. Be sure to communicate these aspects to the interpreting pathologist. Knowledge of these factors can make the difference between a true-negative and a false-negative diagnosis.

Immediate microscopic examination at the time of the aspiration can be helpful, but is not necessary. A high level of diagnostic ability is not required to evaluate for sample adequacy. Examination allows the aspirator to determine if the needle is on target and if adequate material is being obtained and to reposition the needle if necessary on subsequent passes. It can be difficult to define an adequate sample. When assessing whether sufficient material is obtained, the level of clinical suspicion based on physical and mammographic findings, the resistance of the needle, and confidence in aspirating technique should be considered. Aspirates from carcinomas are usually highly cellular while those from fibrocystic nodules are scant and are composed chiefly of fibrofat and only a few ductal cells (Figs. 5-4 through 5-7). Examining the specimen at the time of aspiration also allows one to determine if additional studies requiring special collection methods will be necessary. Toluidine blue O is an excellent quick stain because it requires only a single dropper bottle of stain and can be placed immediately on an alcohol-fixed slide and coverslipped. Following immediate evaluation, the toluidine blue-stained slide can then be placed in a jar of 95% alcohol that further fixes the slide, bleaches the toluidine blue, and allows it to be restained with a Papanicolaou stain for final diagnosis. Many clinicians do not feel comfortable evaluating their own smears for adequacy. Fixing the

UNIVERSITY OF HE... ...E LAU

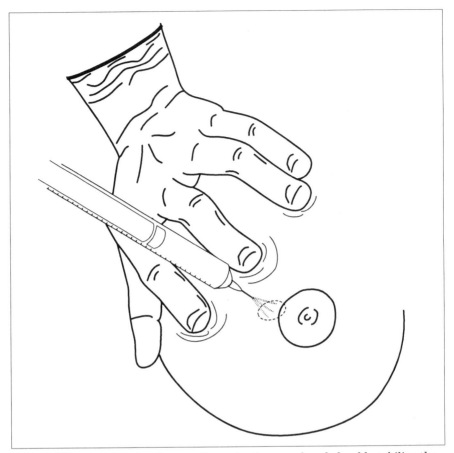

Fig. 5-2. When performing fine needle aspiration, one hand should stabilize the mass between two fingers, while the other directs the needle into multiple areas within the mass.

smears immediately and sending them directly to the laboratory for full evaluation is a perfectly acceptable option. Each lab has its own preference on how it would like to receive the specimen and in what fixative. It is advisable to check with the pathologist.

Occasionally cyst fluid will be obtained by FNA. Because less than 1% of all cysts harbor a malignancy, it is not considered to be cost-effective to send all of these fluids for cytologic evaluation. However, if the fluid obtained appears bloody or necrotic, if a residual mass remains following aspiration, or if the fluid rapidly recurs in 1 to 2 days, the contents of these cysts should be evaluated microscopically. These cysts are more likely to be malignant.

The FNA report is usually signed out with similar terminology to that used in surgical pathology; therefore, a report from a malignant lesion may read *ductal carcinoma,* and from a benign lesion, *fibro-adenoma* or *cells consistent with fibrocystic changes.* Occasionally, the findings may not be definitive and a *suspicious for carcinoma* diagnosis may result. In experienced laboratories, suspicious diag-

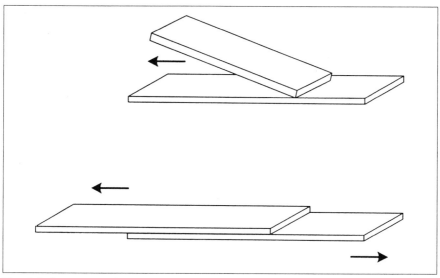

Fig. 5-3. Smears can be prepared by using the edge of a slide *(top)*, or by using the "pull-apart" method *(below)* to evenly spread the aspirated material.

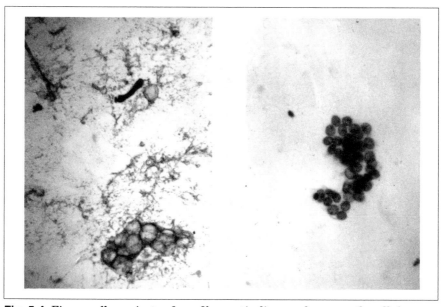

Fig. 5-4. Fine needle aspirates from fibrocystic disease show scantly cellular aspirates with fragments of fibrofat *(left)* and occasional tightly cohesive epithelial cell clusters with nuclei that are uniform in size and shape *(right)*. (Pap, 100× left, 400× right).

noses occur in less than 10% of the cases and often do represent cancers. Thus, a "suspicious" diagnosis should be a meaningful diagnosis and deserves clinical pursuit. Occasionally, *inadequate for diagnosis* may occur and the clinician needs to consider the reason for inadequacy and whether these can be overcome by repeat aspi-

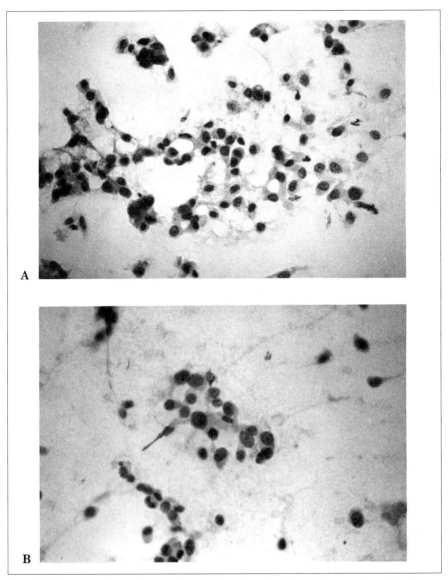

Fig. 5-5. Fine needle aspirates from infiltrating ductal carcinoma show highly cellular specimens (A) containing dyshesive cell groups, and variability in nuclear size and conspicuous nucleoli (B) (Pap, 400×).

ration, or if another diagnostic method is more appropriate. Inadequate specimens are minimized by evaluating specimens at the time of aspiration and by taking corrective action at that time to obtain a better sample.

Advantages

FNA is a simple, safe office procedure that can be performed on palpable masses with little if any discomfort. The advantages of this biopsy method are compared with those of other methods in Table

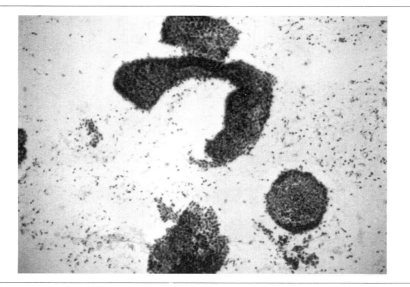

Fig. 5-6. Characteristic cytologic pattern for fibroadenoma with large branching sheets of epithelial cells and naked nuclei in the background. (Pap, 250×).

5-3. Some nonpalpable lesions can be aspirated under mammographic or ultrasound guidance as well (see Chap. 6). A small bruise at the aspiration site is the only significant complication. Tumor seeding along the needle track is extremely rare, estimated at 0.005% (1 : 20,000). Multiple lesions can be easily aspirated in the same office visit, and results can be obtained that same day. By performing multiple passes and redirecting the needle during each pass one can sample different areas within the mass to obtain a truly representative specimen. Sensitivity and specificity are reported to be 96% and 94% respectively for the diagnosis of carcinoma, but must be combined with mammographic and clinical findings for accurate use (Fig. 5-8). The ease and accuracy of this biopsy method allows masses to be sampled immediately, reducing the anxiety associated with "wait and watch" clinical follow-up. A malignant diagnosis allows the patient and physician to discuss treatment options preoperatively. Definitive treatment can take place on the basis of an FNA diagnosis, eliminating the need for surgical biopsy or frozen section (Fig. 5-9). A benign diagnosis does not preclude the need for clinical follow-up, but provides further reassurance that a mass is benign and, in many instances, can obviate surgery.

Disadvantages
FNA cannot distinguish in situ from invasive carcinomas. In addition, not all pathologists are equally proficient or comfortable interpreting breast FNAs. Common causes of false-negative diagnoses are errors in needle placement, highly sclerotic cancers such as infiltrating lobular carcinoma, and uncommon, well-differentiated subtypes such as tubular or papillary carcinomas. False-positive

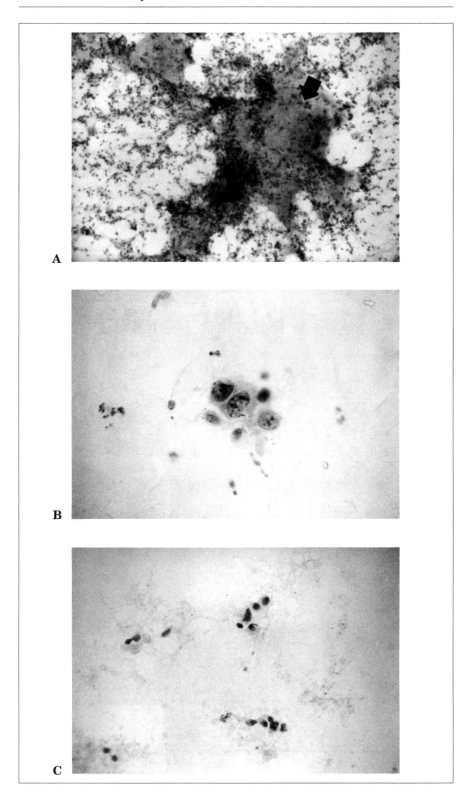

Table 5-3. Relative advantages of various biopsy methods

	Type of biopsy			
	Fine needle aspiration	12-gauge core	14-gauge core	Excisional
Office procedure	Yes	Yes	Yes	No
Pain	+	+++	++	+++
Hemorrhage	+	++	+	++
Tumor seeding	Rare	Possible	Possible	Rare
Wide sampling	++	0	++ if multiple biopsies performed	+++
Ability to distinguish invasion	No	Yes	Yes	Yes
Easy interpretation	+	++	++	+++
Cost-effectiveness	+++	++	++	+

+ = minimal; ++ = moderate; +++ = greatest.

diagnoses are rare when they are interpreted by experienced cyto-pathologists. Slightly more common are false suspicious diagnoses that may be due to fibrocystic changes with much epithelial hyperplasia, proliferative fibroadenomas, or hyperplasia due to pregnancy or lactation.

Cutting Needle Biopsy

Large core biopsies have traditionally been performed with 12-gauge cutting needles. Local anesthesia is injected subcutaneously at the site, the skin is incised with a scalpel, and the cutting needle is inserted. Recently, thinner 14-gauge needles attached to a rapid-fire biopsy gun similar to those commonly used in the prostate have been employed. Both methods obtain a solid core of tissue for histologic diagnosis. Pathologists are generally most proficient at examining this type of specimen. The biopsy specimen should be fixed in formalin. However, unlike FNA, sampling is not as widely representative because the needle only retrieves the single spot that it penetrates; therefore, multiple biopsies are recommended with the rapid-fire gun. Multiple biopsies are not practical with the traditional cutting needle biopsy because it is relatively painful and induces much local hemorrhage. Tumor seeding along with needle track is also a concern with these wider-gauge needles, and excision

Fig. 5-7. Aspiration biopsy cytology can distinguish special forms of breast cancer: Mucinous carcinoma (A) contains pools of mucin in background *(arrow)*; medullary carcinoma (B) is characterized by large pleomorphic cells with a sprinkling of lymphocytes in the background; and a scant aspirate with cells arranged linearly denotes lobular carcinoma (C) (Pap, A, C = 250×, B = 400×).

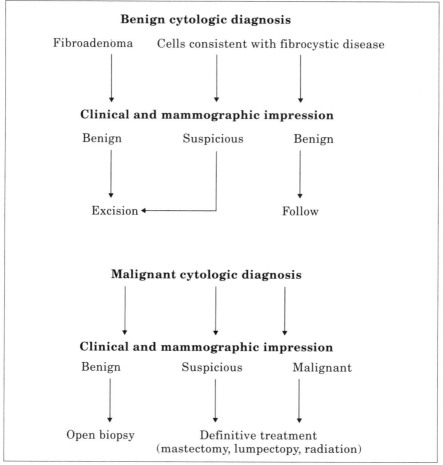

Fig. 5-8. Use of fine needle aspiration in clinical problem solving. The cytologic diagnosis should be correlated with clinical and mammographic information for optimal clinical decision making.

of the track may be recommended when a malignant tumor is diagnosed.

Excisional Biopsy

Excisional biopsy is considered the gold standard because it removes the entire lesion for histologic examination. If the lesion is not palpable, mammographic localization must be performed (see Chap. 6). A curvilinear incision following the normal contour of the breast gives the best cosmetic result. The entire lesion should be removed with a surrounding rim of normal tissue and, if the latter is wide enough, it is equivalent to a lumpectomy for breast cancer treatment. Because a large specimen is usually obtained, portions of the lesion will be sent by the pathologist for special prognostic studies in addition to routine histology. The biopsy specimen should always be sent

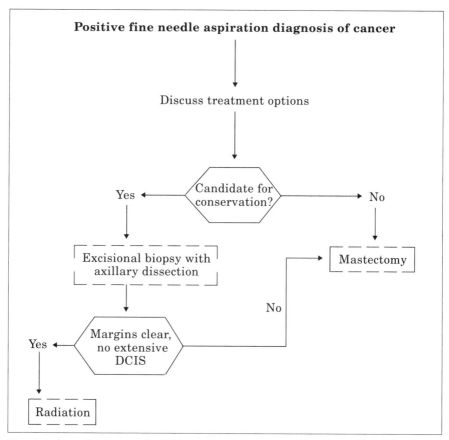

Positive fine needle aspiration diagnosis of cancer

Discuss treatment options

Candidate for conservation?

Yes

No

Excisional biopsy with axillary dissection

Mastectomy

No

Margins clear, no extensive DCIS

Yes

Radiation

Fig. 5-9. A malignant cytologic diagnosis of cancer is useful for patients undergoing mastectomy or breast-conserving therapy and does not require frozen-section confirmation. DCIS = ductal carcinoma in situ.

fresh and unfixed to the laboratory so the pathologist can triage it appropriately. Keeping the specimen cool on ice (but not frozen) can be beneficial if a delay in transport is anticipated.

Excisional biopsy carries the typical surgical risks of potential wound infection and hemorrhage, and the presence of a scar postoperatively. Because this biopsy is usually performed by a surgeon in an outpatient surgical suite, the costs are not insignificant. Because the vast majority of breast masses are benign and many women have frequent and multiple breast masses, the cost and surgical risks can be disadvantages.

Understanding the Surgical Pathology Report

The written report is the pathologist's vehicle for telling the clinician what it is she or he is seeing under the microscope and what that means about the patient and her disease.

When the Diagnosis Is Cancer

A good surgical pathology report should include the following:

1. **Type of cancer** (ductal, lobular, special type). Certain types of breast cancer carry specific prognostic significance, as indicated in Chap. 3. For example, lobular cancers are more frequently multifocal and bilateral and medullary and tubular carcinomas have a better prognosis than the usual ductal carcinoma.
2. **Presence of invasion.** Distinguishing in situ from invasive disease is an important prognostic indicator. The presence of vascular or lymphatic invasion within the tumor may be an indication for radiation.
3. **Size of cancer.** Size is important in staging.
4. **Grade of cancer.** Tumor grade is a method of expressing tumor differentiation for ductal carcinomas and indicates prognosis. The most common breast tumor-grading system is the Scarff-Bloom-Richardson system in which three features (the degree of tubule formation, the frequency of mitoses, and nuclear pleomorphism) are each assigned a score from 1 to 3. The score of each of the three features is added together for a final sum that will range from 3 to 9. A tumor with a sum of 3, 4, or 5 is considered to be grade I or well differentiated; a sum of 6 or 7 is grade II or moderately differentiated; and a poorly differentiated tumor will be a grade III with a sum of 8 or 9. High-grade tumors behave more aggressively than low-grade tumors and carry a poorer prognosis.
5. **Presence of in situ cancer, type, and extent.** The comedo type of ductal carcinoma in situ is a more aggressive form than other types. When carcinoma in situ is considered extensive, breast conserving therapy may not be an option.
6. **Involvement of margins.** The surgical margins of resection must be free of in situ and invasive cancer for the excision to be considered therapeutic. If the margins are not free of tumor, further surgery is usually indicated. This may be another, wider excision or a mastectomy.

Special Studies

The most important prognostic factors are generally considered to be tumor size, nodal status, and hormone receptor status. Additional special studies (listed below) are performed routinely to help identify breast cancers with a poor prognosis so that therapy can be individualized and those patients can be treated and followed more aggressively. These studies reflect medicine's increased understanding of breast cancer biology. Investigational work is ongoing to evaluate their effectiveness. Although these studies can be performed most easily on an excisional biopsy because of the abundant tissue obtained, they also can be performed on FNAs and core biopsies.

1. **Estrogen and progesterone receptors.** The presence of these

receptors helps determine whether a patient is a candidate for hormonal therapy. Tumors from older patients are more often positive than those from younger patients, probably because the receptors in the younger patients are bound with endogenous hormones and are therefore not available for measurement or for therapeutic manipulation. In general, hormone receptor-positive tumors have a better prognosis.

2. **DNA ploidy.** The amount of DNA present in the tumor can help to predict prognosis. Aneuploid tumors, those with an abnormal amount of DNA, indicate a more unfavorable outcome than diploid tumors. Diploid tumors may have a lower probability of developing drug-resistant mutations when the total tumor cell burden is small and any metastases may remain dormant for a long time.

3. **Synthetic-phase fraction (SPF or %S-phase), and Ki-67.** These measurements estimate the tumor's proliferative component. High-proliferative components tend to have a poor prognosis. Synthetic-phase fraction is a measurement of the number of cells in the synthetic phase of cell cycle. It is an excellent prognosticator in node-negative patients. Ki-67 is a nuclear protein associated with cell proliferation within all phases of the cell cycle except the resting phase. Ki-67 correlates with SPF and mitotic counts and is more likely to be associated with aneuploid tumors, high histologic grade, and estrogen receptor/progesterone receptor (ER/PR) negativity.

4. **Her-2-Neu oncogene.** Overexpression of this gene's product correlates with a shorter relapse time and with shorter overall survival in node-positive breast cancer patients, although it is not predictive in node-negative patients. However, it can be expressed in certain types of ductal carcinoma in situ, particularly the comedo subtype, and may indicate that these patients are at risk for relapse.

5. **Cathepsin D.** This enzyme is thought to assist cell migration and metastasis by digesting basement membrane and extracellular matrix. Overexpression was originally believed to help predict risk of recurrence and survival in node-negative patients, although this is now being questioned.

6. **Epidermal growth factor receptor (EGFR).** This receptor binds a protein involved in normal cell growth. Amplification of the EGFR gene is accompanied by increased expression. EGFR-positive patients have a shorter disease-free interval and poorer overall survival than those who are EGFR negative. This study can help stratify estrogen receptor-negative patients into poor and good prognostic categories.

When the Diagnosis Is Benign

The most important information the pathologist can convey is the fact that cancer is not present. Most benign breast masses are due to fibrocystic changes, which include a variety of histologic findings. The only two of significance are atypical ductal or lobular hyperplasia because they increase (4 to 5 times) the patient's risk of developing a subsequent invasive breast cancer (see Chap. 3). In a patient with a mother or sister with breast cancer, the finding of atypical hyperplasia will increase her risk 10 times, or equal to that of a patient with carcinoma in situ.

Suggested Reading

Clark GM, et al. How to integrate steroid hormone receptor, flow cytometric, and other prognostic information in regard to primary breast cancer. *Cancer* 71:2157–2162, 1993.

Hutter RVP. The role of the pathologist in breast cancer management. *Cancer* 66:1363–1372, 1990.

Joensuu H, et al. DNA index and S-phase fraction and their combination as prognostic factors in operable ductal breast carcinoma. *Cancer* 66:331–340, 1990.

Kline TS, and Kline IK. *Guides to Clinical Aspiration Biopsy: Breast.* New York: Igaku-Shoin Medical Publishers, 1989.

Langmuir VK, et al. Fine needle aspiration cytology in the management of palpable benign and malignant breast disease: Correlation with clinical and mammographic findings. *Acta Cytologica* 33:93–98, 1988.

McGuire WL, et al. How to use prognostic factors in axillary node-negative breast cancer patients. *J Natl Cancer Inst* 82:1006–1015, 1990.

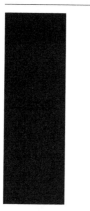

Evaluation of
Clinical Problems

The Occult Lesion

Karen K. Lindfors

Screening mammography is important in the detection of early stage, clinically occult breast cancer, but it is only the first step in the diagnosis of this disease. Many ambiguous abnormalities are seen on screening mammograms. For this reason a woman who has undergone a screening study may receive a call or letter asking her to return to the radiologist's office for additional mammographic views or ultrasound. In turn, the referring clinician may get a frantic call from the woman who is alarmed about having to return. Such women should be reassured that a return visit does not mean that she has breast cancer; it simply means that the radiologist wishes to clarify what was seen on the initial screening study. Only about 1 out of every 10 women recalled will prove to have a carcinoma.

If a woman attends a radiology facility at which screening mammography is immediately followed by any views or studies necessary for clarification, she may become similarly anxious if asked to undergo such additional procedures. Women should be informed that a mammographic screening *begins* with two views of each breast and that additional views or ultrasound are frequently necessary.

Clarification of Screening Mammography Results

One of the caveats of mammography is that lesions must be visualized in two projections to be considered real. For example, superimposed normal breast structures in one view can appear as a mass, which could cause the radiologist concern that the lesion is obscured by overlying parenchyma in the other view. This situation can be clarified by performing mammography from other angles or by performing spot compression views over the area of concern (Fig. 6-1). Spot compression is accomplished by using a small round compression paddle that exerts greater compressive force over the underlying tissue. If the questionable mass is the result of superimposed normal structures, these structures will be spread apart to reveal normal breast architecture when spot compression is used.

Although most women have reasonably symmetric breast parenchyma, at least 3% have areas of asymmetric, but histologically normal, tissue. This can confuse the mammographer, but spot compres-

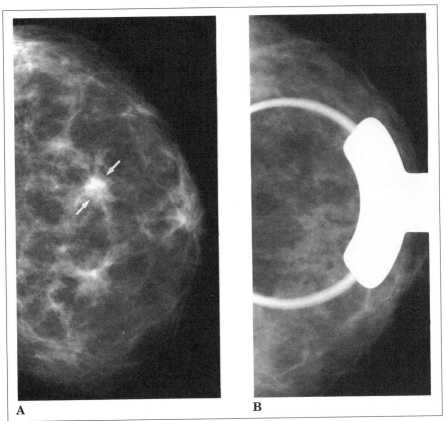

Fig. 6-1. Craniocaudal view of the left breast (A) shows a possible ill-defined mass *(arrows)* in the central part of the breast. Spot compression (B) over the questionable area spreads the tissues and shows normal architecture. The "mass" was the result of a superimposition of normal structures.

sion also can usually resolve this question by spreading the tissues apart and demonstrating normal architecture (Fig. 6-2). Areas of asymmetry are significant only if a palpable mass is associated. It is important for the clinician to examine carefully the area identified on the mammogram as asymmetric.

Additional information about masses or calcifications seen on screening mammograms can be gained by performing magnification views. Magnification views provide a more accurate assessment of the margins of masses and the morphology of microcalcifications. Such information is very useful in deciding whether a biopsy is warranted.

Ultrasound also can be useful in problem solving. When a well-circumscribed mass is seen on screening mammography, it may represent a simple cyst. Cysts are easily diagnosed using high-frequency hand-held ultrasound targeted to the lesion seen on the films. Ultrasound can also be used to diagnose a cyst when the borders of

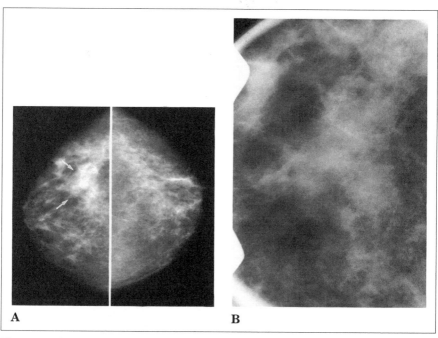

Fig. 6-2. Bilateral craniocaudal mammograms (A) demonstrate asymmetric breast tissue in the lateral aspect of the right breast *(arrows)*. Because of a questionable mass in this area, a spot compression film (B) was obtained that demonstrated normal parenchymal architecture in the area of asymmetry. No mass was identified. (From Lindfors K. Breast Imaging. In WE Brant and CA Helms (eds), *Fundamentals of Diagnostic Radiology.* Baltimore: Williams & Wilkins, 1994.)

a mass are obscured by overlying breast tissue on the mammogram. *Ultrasound, however, is not useful in distinguishing benign solid masses from those that are malignant.*

About 10% of women undergoing screening mammography will require further assessment with additional mammographic views or ultrasound. Of those, less than one-third will be recommended for biopsy.

Understanding the Breast Imaging Report

Attempts are being made by the American College of Radiology (ACR) to create national standards for mammography reporting. Adoption of the ACR's Breast Imaging Reporting and Database (BIRD) System allows radiologists to communicate the mammography report to the referring clinician in a clear and concise manner. Standardized terminology is recommended. The mammography report should include a statement about the overall composition of the breast, a description of any lesions or abnormalities, and a final assessment. Those radiologists who have not yet adopted the BIRD System frequently employ a similar format although their terminology may vary.

Breast Composition

Understanding the overall composition of the breasts allows the clinician to gauge the sensitivity of the mammogram. If the breast tissue is completely replaced by fat, detection of a lesion by mammography will be facilitated (Fig. 6-3). If, however, the breasts are heterogeneously dense (Fig. 6-4), it may be more difficult to visualize a lesion. When the breasts are extremely dense (formerly called dysplastic), as shown in Fig. 6-5, parenchymal abnormalities are fre-

Fig. 6-3. Left mediolateral oblique view of a normal fatty replaced breast. Lesions are easiest to see in this type of breast.

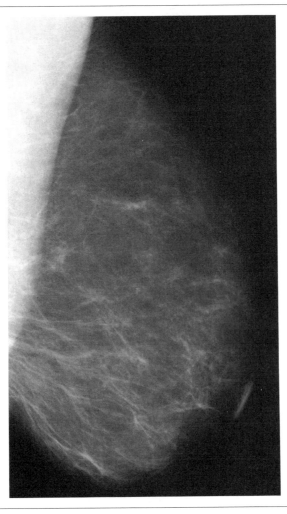

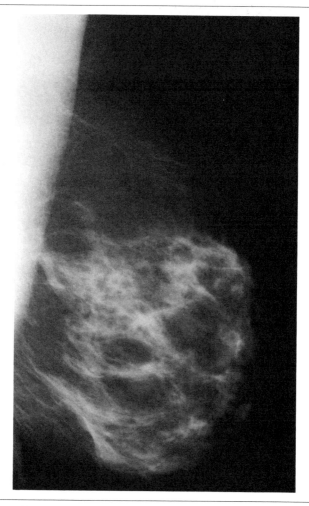

Fig. 6-4. Normal left mediolateral oblique mammogram showing heterogeneously dense breast tissue. Small lesions could be obscured in this type of breast.

quently obscured and thus the sensitivity of mammography is lowered. However, because calcifications can be visualized, mammography is still useful in women with extremely dense breasts.

Masses

When a mass is found on mammography, clinicians will find the description of the margins to be most helpful in assessing the probability of malignancy (Table 6-1).

Spiculated Margins

Spiculated margins (formerly called stellate margins) will confer the highest probability of malignancy on a mass (Fig. 6-6). Surgical or

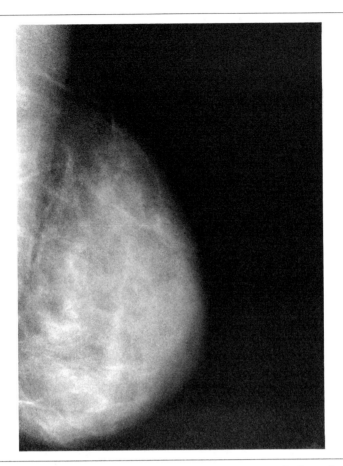

Fig. 6-5. Normal left mediolateral oblique view of an extremely dense breast. The sensitivity of mammography is lower in women with dense breasts since masses are often obscured.

Table 6-1. Differential diagnosis of breast masses based on margin characteristics

Type of margin seen on mammogram		
Spiculated	Ill defined	Well defined
Cancer	Fibrocystic change	Cyst
Fat necrosis or scar	Cancer	Fibroadenoma
Complex sclerosing lesion	Hematoma	Lymph node
(radial scar)	Abscess	Focal fibrosis
		Cancer

other posttraumatic scarring can also appear as a spiculated mass, but careful correlation with the patient's history and comparison with previous films should allow a diagnosis in such cases. Complex sclerosing lesions or radial scars can also appear as spiculated masses; mammographic differentiation of this benign entity from malignancy is impossible.

Ill-Defined Margins

When the margins of a lesion are described as ill defined or indistinct there is a significant chance of malignancy, but fibrocystic changes, hematomas, and abscesses commonly have this appearance as well (Fig. 6-7).

Sometimes the margins of a lesion may be difficult to assess because of overlying parenchyma (Fig. 6-8). Although additional

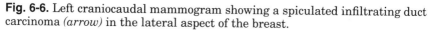

Fig. 6-6. Left craniocaudal mammogram showing a spiculated infiltrating duct carcinoma *(arrow)* in the lateral aspect of the breast.

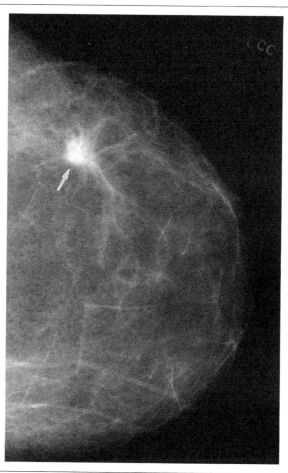

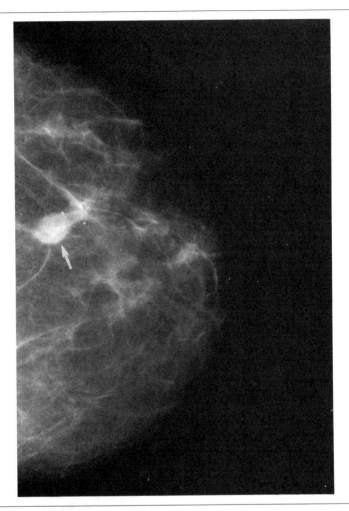

Fig. 6-7. A mass with ill-defined margins *(arrow)* representing a hematoma is seen on this left craniocaudal view. The patient had undergone a recent excisional biopsy of fibroadenoma in this location.

mammographic views may help clarify the appearance of such a mass, it is frequently impossible to gain a view of the mass free of overlying tissue.

Well-Defined Margins

Masses with well-defined margins (i.e., well-circumscribed masses) are least likely to represent cancer (Fig. 6-9). Cysts, fibroadenomas, focal fibrosis, and intramammary lymph nodes are some commonly seen well-circumscribed masses. Up to 5% of breast cancers, however, also can present as well-circumscribed masses. The radiologist must take this into consideration when evaluating this type of lesion (Fig. 6-10). If the mass is homogeneously dense and does

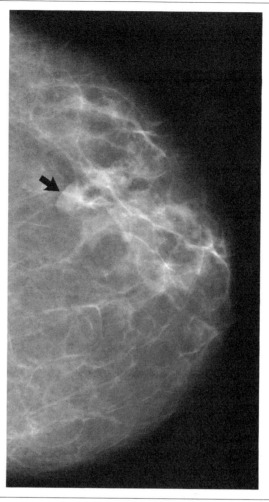

Fig. 6-8. Left craniocaudal view showing a well-circumscribed mass along the posterior border *(arrow)*, obscured anteriorly by overlying parenchyma. The mass was a fibroadenoma at biopsy.

not contain fat, the lesion's size will in part determine the radiologist's next step. If the mass is large enough to be visualized by ultrasound (about 4–5 mm in diameter) that usually will be done next. Ultrasound can distinguish simple cysts, which are virtually never malignant, from noncystic masses. If a cyst is diagnosed, nothing more need be done. If the lesion is not a simple cyst, its size will again be important in deciding whether to biopsy or to follow the patient. Most mammographers will recommend a period of follow-up for well-circumscribed masses that are under 8 to 10 mm in diameter. Such lesions have a low probability of malignancy (less than 1%).

Generally a follow-up mammogram of the affected breast will be

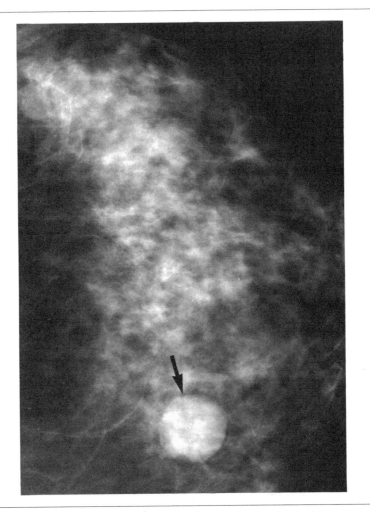

Fig. 6-9. A 2-cm clinically occult well-circumscribed mass *(arrow)* is seen on this left craniocaudal mammogram. At ultrasound this mass was a simple cyst.

recommended 4 to 6 months after the first study. If that examination demonstrates no interval change, a bilateral mammogram will be performed at the one-year anniversary of the first exam and then annually thereafter for at least 4 years. If a well-circumscribed mass is larger than 10 to 15 mm in diameter, biopsy is often recommended to rule out a well-circumscribed cancer.

If there are multiple bilateral well-defined masses, no matter what their size, a benign diagnosis is also likely. Both cysts and fibroadenomas can present as such. The appearance of such a mammogram is usually a surprise because nothing has been felt on physical examination and yet the breasts have a bizarre mammographic appearance with many masses (Fig. 6-11).

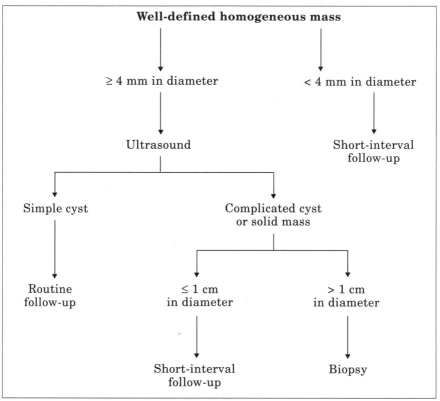

Fig. 6-10. Decision tree for the evaluation of a well-circumscribed, homogenous mass that is discovered on mammography.

Density

The density of a mass seen on mammography is significant only if the mass contains fat. All fat-containing masses are benign. Fat appears as a lucent or dark area on mammography. The most commonly seen fat-containing mass is an *intramammary lymph node* (Fig. 6-12). Such nodes typically appear on mammogram with a fatty center or a fatty notch; these lucent areas represent fat in the hilus of the node. Intramammary lymph nodes are generally located in the lateral half of the breast, usually in the upper outer quadrant (Fig. 6-13). Other fat-containing benign breast masses include lipomas, oil cysts and other forms of fat necrosis, galactoceles, and hamartomas (Fig. 6-14).

Calcifications

Calcifications are often seen in the breast. They are most commonly a benign finding and will not always be reported. Benign calcifications are usually larger than those associated with malignancy and are more regular in shape, often round and smooth. Some benign calcifications have characteristic appearances, which allows their

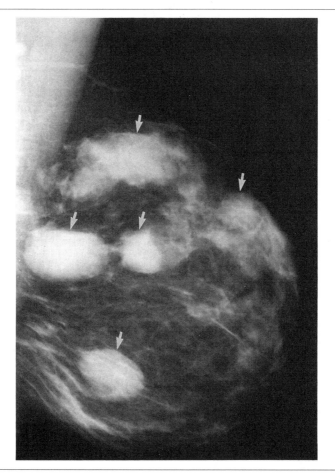

Fig. 6-11. Left mediolateral oblique view showing multiple large round masses *(arrows)*. The patient was totally asymptomatic. The differential diagnosis was multiple cysts versus multiple fibroadenomas.

differentiation from malignant calcifications (Fig. 6-15). Coarse, pop-cornlike calcifications (Fig. 6-15A) are typical for an involuting fibro-adenoma. Parallel tracks of calcium are noted in vascular calcifica-tion (Fig. 6-15B). Eggshell calcifications are seen in cysts or oil cysts (Fig. 6-15C). The term *milk of calcium* refers to sedimented calcium within the fluid of benign microcysts; such calcifications change in appearance from one mammographic view to another. On lateral films milk of calcium calcifications appear as lines or menisci, but on craniocaudal films they appear as smudges (Fig. 6-16). Lucent-cen-tered calcifications are also benign (Fig. 6-17). They can be seen in the skin, in areas of fat necrosis, or in ducts. Large rod-shaped cal-cifications pointing toward the nipple can be seen in mammary duct ectasia (Fig. 6-18).

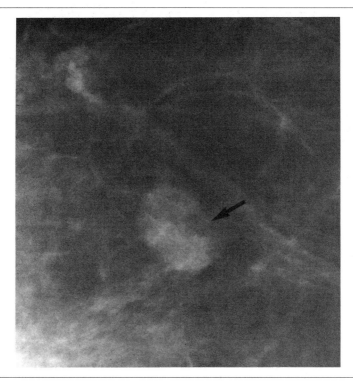

Fig. 6-12. Magnification view of an intramammary lymph node. Note the fatty hilus *(arrow)* that appears as a lucent or darker area within the node.

True calcifications must be distinguished from artifacts. *Artifacts* can occur from dust on the film or defects in the emulsion of the film. Artifacts can also be due to deodorant, powders, or creams on the patient's skin, which is why patients are asked not to use such substances before mammography.

Classically *malignant calcifications* are heterogeneous in size and shape. Malignant calcifications are always small (less than .5 mm in diameter), are usually numerous, and are clustered within a small volume of tissue. They can be linear or branched, especially when associated with the comedo type of ductal carcinoma in situ (Fig. 6-19). More granular-shaped calcifications are seen in the noncomedo varieties of ductal carcinoma in situ (Fig. 6-20). Over 50% of all breast carcinomas seen mammographically have associated microcalcifications. Over 70% of noninvasive breast carcinomas are manifest by calcifications alone. Even when a suspicious cluster of microcalcifications does not have an associated soft tissue mass, it should still be biopsied.

Less than 25% of all occult cancers will present with typical malignant calcifications. Almost an equal number of cancers will be discovered from biopsies of calcifications that are less specific in

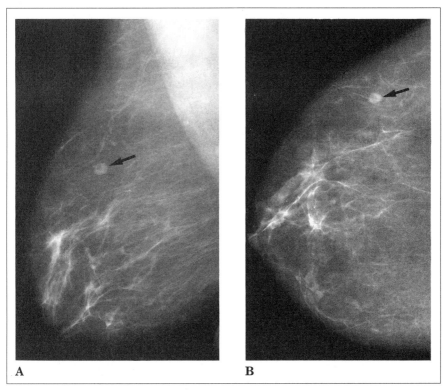

Fig. 6-13. Right mediolateral oblique (A) and craniocaudal (B) mammograms showing a typical intramammary lymph node *(arrows)* at about the 10 o'clock position. Note the fatty center of the node.

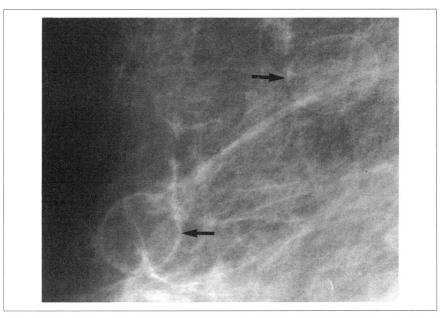

Fig. 6-14. Magnified view showing two oil cysts *(arrows)*. These are lucent (fat density) masses surrounded by thin capsules.

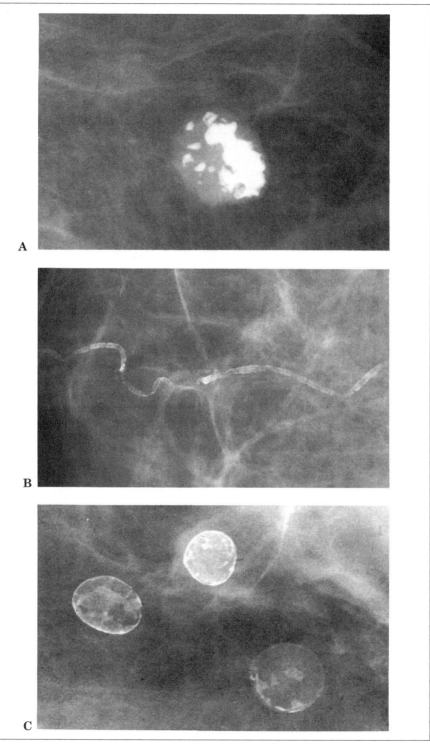

Fig. 6-15. Typical benign calcifications. Coarse, popcornlike calcifications (A) are typical of an involuting fibroadenoma. Vascular calcifications (B) are a frequent finding in older women. Eggshell calcifications (C) have formed in the walls of these oil cysts.

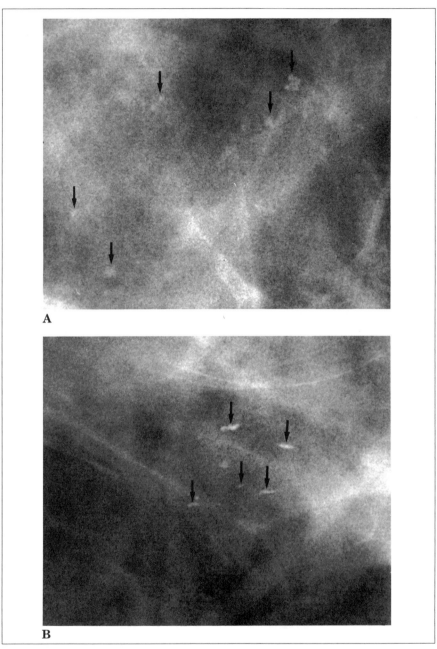

Fig. 6-16. Magnification views of benign "milk of calcium" within microcysts. On the craniocaudal views (A) the calcifications are seen as tiny ill-defined smudges *(arrows)*, but on the lateral view (B) the calcifications *(arrows)* appear linear because the meniscus of calcium containing fluid is being viewed from the side.

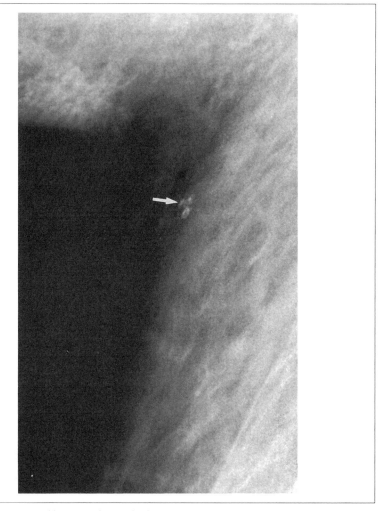

Fig. 6-17. A group of benign skin calcifications with lucent centers *(arrow)* are seen in the inframammary fold.

appearance. Such calcifications are indeterminate, but must be biopsied because malignancy cannot be excluded. The probability of finding cancer from a biopsy of an indeterminate cluster of microcalcifications is about 25% to 30%.

Other Mammographic Findings

Architectural distortion also may be reported on mammogram. In this case, although no mass is visible, spiculations may be seen radiating from a point or there may be focal retraction in the parenchyma (Fig. 6-21). Such findings must be considered suspicious for malig-

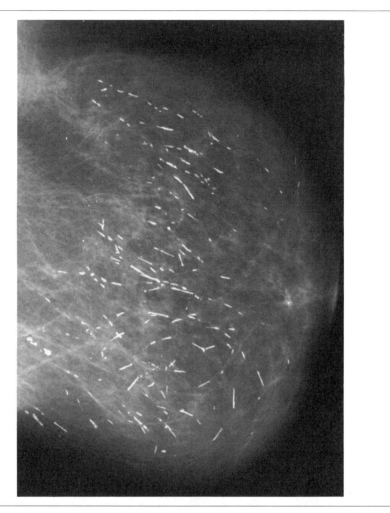

Fig. 6-18. The diffuse, large rod-shaped calcifications seen on this left craniocaudal view are benign; they are the typical calcifications of mammary duct ectasia.

nancy, although they also can represent scarring, fat necrosis, or a radial scar.

A change in the appearance of the mammogram when compared to previous ones may be reported. The majority of such changes will be benign, but the appearance of a new mass or enlargement of an existing mass is cause for further work-up (i.e., ultrasound, fine needle aspiration, or biopsy). Similarly, the appearance of a new cluster of microcalcifications often prompts a biopsy.

Asymmetric tissue may be identified mammographically and should prompt a careful physical examination by the clinician to determine whether there is an associated suspicious palpable abnormality. If such a palpable abnormality exists fine needle aspiration

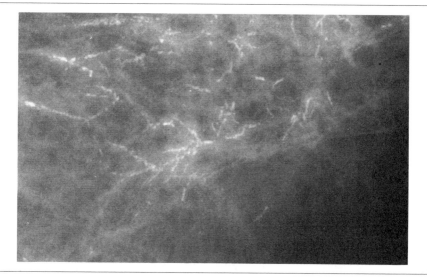

Fig. 6-19. Typical fine linear or "casting" malignant calcifications seen in comedo-type ductal carcinoma in situ.

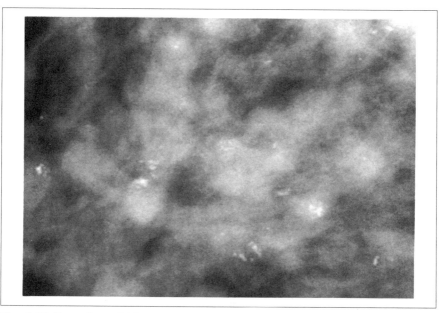

Fig. 6-20. Irregular calcifications that are pleomorphic and more granular in appearance. Such malignant calcifications often are seen in noncomedo-type ductal carcinoma in situ.

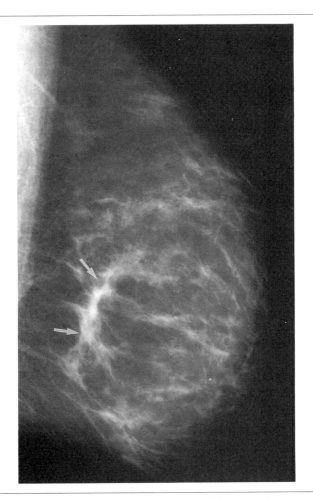

Fig. 6-21. Architectural distortion *(arrows)* is noted deep in the breast on this left mediolateral oblique view. At biopsy this was invasive lobular carcinoma.

or biopsy should be performed. If normal tissue is felt on examination, it is safe to follow and not biopsy the patient.

A diffuse increase in the density of the breast associated with skin thickening can indicate inflammatory carcinoma, postradiotherapy sequelae, diffuse mastitis, or edema (Fig. 6-22). Correlation with history and physical examination should narrow the diagnostic possibilities. Hormone replacement therapy can cause a bilateral increase in the density of the breast parenchyma but is not associated with skin thickening (Fig. 6-23). It can, however, obscure previously seen or new masses.

Other findings, such as dilated ducts or enlarged veins, are non-specific and if unassociated with other abnormalities are not usually considered significant.

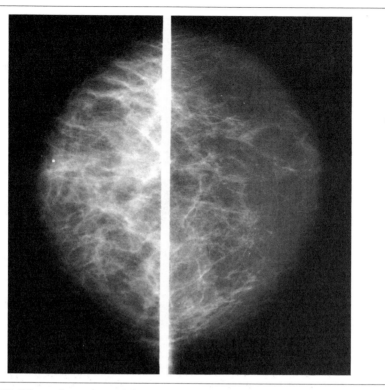

Fig. 6-22. Bilateral craniocaudal mammograms of a woman with right inflammatory carcinoma of the breast. Note the diffuse increase in density of the right breast compared with the left. Skin thickening could be seen on the right when a bright light was used.

Lesion Location

The location of any lesion described in the mammography report should be specified. The American College of Radiology suggests that the clock-face position, as well as an indication of depth within the breast, be used to describe location. This approach provides a more exact description than does the general quadrant location, thus facilitating correlation with the physical examination.

When orthogonal views of the breast (i.e., craniocaudal, straight, or 90-degree lateral) are available, it is usually simple to locate the lesion three dimensionally within the breast; however, a straight lateral view generally is not taken during screening mammography. The oblique view is the preferred second view. Because this view is taken at an obliquity, which can vary from patient to patient (usually between 45 and 60 degrees), it becomes more difficult to locate a lesion with reference to the clock face.

If the viewer hangs the craniocaudal view next to the oblique view with the nipple pointed in the same direction and at the same level

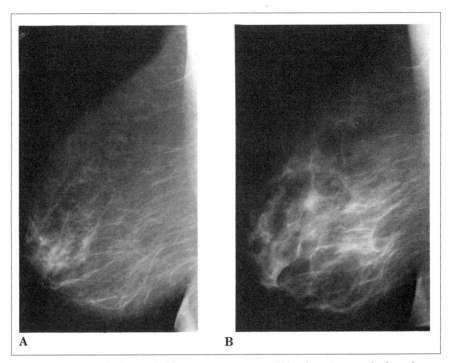

Fig. 6-23. Left mediolateral oblique mammogram (A) taken 2 years before the subsequent film (B) that shows a diffuse increase in the parenchymal density of the breast without skin thickening. The patient had been placed on hormone replacement therapy in the period between the films.

it can be relatively easy to determine the approximate location of this lesion on a 90-degree lateral view and then to triangulate to the clock face. If an arrow is drawn from the lesion on the craniocaudal view through its location on the oblique view, the arrow will point to the lesion's location on a straight lateral view (Fig. 6-24). For example, if a lesion is located medially on a craniocaudal view and is seen above the nipple level on the oblique view, it will be located superiorly on a lateral view.

At times a potential abnormality seen well in one view can be difficult to locate in the second view. Several possible explanations for this occurrence include the following:

1. The lesion may be located in an area not imaged in the second view. For example, lesions located in the axillary tail of the breast are frequently not seen on standard craniocaudal views. Special views are needed to image such lesions.

2. The abnormality may be located in the skin. Skin lesions, such as calcifications or moles, can be seen en face in one projection, making them appear to be in the breast (Fig. 6-25A). In the second mammographic projection the lesion may not be visualized because it is within the skin that is tangent to the x-ray beam

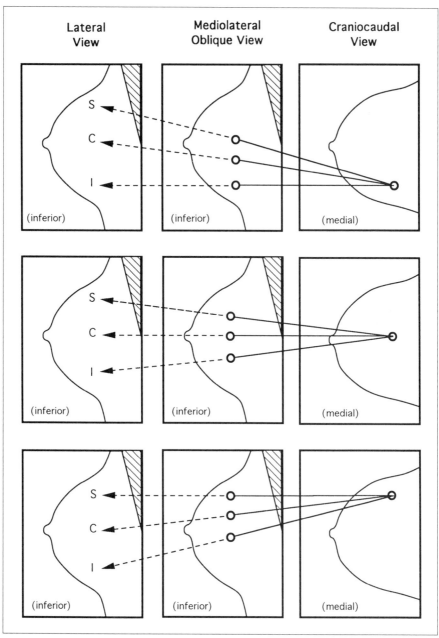

Fig. 6-24. Method for determining the location of a lesion in the 90-degree orthogonal plane. The craniocaudal view should be hung next to the mediolateral oblique view with the nipple pointed in the same direction and at the same level. If an arrow is drawn from the lesion on the craniocaudal view to the lesion as seen on the oblique view, it will point to the location of the lesion on a hypothetical straight (90 degrees) lateral. This information can be helpful in determining the exact location of the lesion in the breast. (Adapted from Sickles EA. Practical solutions to common mammographic problems: Tailoring the examination. *AJR* 151:31, 1988.)

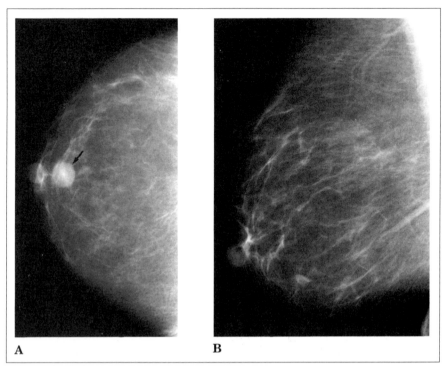

A   B

Fig. 6-25. A well-circumscribed round mass *(arrow)* is seen just deep to the nipple in this right craniocaudal view (A). The mass "disappears" on the mediolateral oblique view (B). Illumination with a bright light showed the mass, which was a sebaceous cyst, to be in the skin inferior to the nipple.

(Fig. 6-25B). Using a bright light to illuminate the skin of the breast will usually resolve this problem by demonstrating the lesion.

3. The abnormality may be obscured by overlying dense tissue in the second projection. In this case it is helpful for the observer to focus on the area most likely to contain the lesion. This is done by measuring the distance from the lesion to an imaginary line that is tangential to the nipple and, in the mediolateral oblique view, parallel to the pectoralis major muscle. Once this distance is determined the observer can measure the same distance back from a similar imaginary line on the second view to determine the axis in which the lesion should lie (Fig. 6-26). Additional views for clarification can then be taken.

4. Most commonly a potential abnormality is seen well in one view but not in the other because the abnormality does not represent a true lesion, but rather is the result of a superimposition of structures in one view. In the second view these structures are separated, hence no lesion is seen. Remember the important caveat of

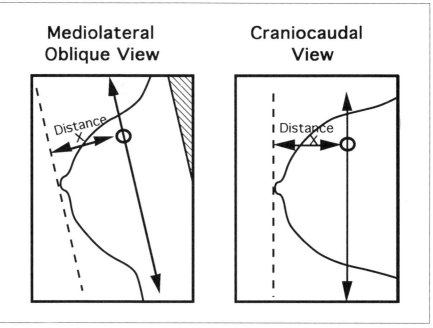

Fig. 6-26. Method for locating a lesion in two mammographic views. In both views the lesion should be located along a line that is the same distance posterior to the reference lines *(dashed)*. Reference lines *(dashed)* are drawn parallel to the pectoralis major muscle through the nipple on the oblique view and tangential to the nipple on the craniocaudal view.

mammographic interpretation: *In order to be considered a true lesion, the abnormality must be seen in two views.*

The Final Assessment

The final assessment of the findings is the most important part of the breast imaging report. It contains the synthesis of all the information gathered by the radiologist. The imaging findings are correlated with the patient's history and physical examination to determine both the probability of malignancy (Table 6-2) and the recommendation for future action.

Table 6-2. Probability that a lesion is malignant*

Assessment	Probability of malignancy
Negative or benign	0%
Short-interval follow-up suggested	0.5–2%
Suspicious, biopsy should be considered	25–30%
High probability of breast cancer	98–99%

*Based on final assessment given in the mammography report.

Knowledge of the patient's history is helpful in assessing the probability of malignancy or likely diagnosis of a particular mammographic finding. The risk of malignancy is much greater in a 60-year-old woman than it is in a 30-year-old woman. A woman with a personal or family history of breast cancer is at greater risk for malignancy, and the interpretation of her mammographic findings should be tailored accordingly. Other information, such as previous surgical biopsies or hormone intake, must also be taken into account when interpreting breast imaging studies.

Most radiology practices use a history form (see Appendix B) to obtain information on a woman's breast health, but communication from the referring physician about specific indications for the examination is also useful. This communication should include clear information regarding the breast physical examination findings. All of this information helps the radiologist render the most accurate assessment of what is found on the imaging studies.

If the final assessment of breast imaging studies is reported as negative, the next screening mammogram should be obtained as established guidelines recommend (see Chap. 4). The same plan is recommended when unequivocal benign findings are present. Such findings are reported only if they are distinctive and might be confused with more suspicious findings by those who are not experienced at mammographic interpretation.

When short-interval follow-up is suggested (i.e., 4–6 months) the lesion is highly likely to be benign. The radiologist anticipates no change in the lesion on the follow-up study, but there is still a finite, albeit very low, probability that the lesion is malignant. Short-interval follow-up is an accepted alternative to biopsy for such lesions, and most patients prefer this approach when counseled that their risk of malignancy is about 1 in 100. If, however, the patient is uncomfortable waiting for follow-up, a biopsy can certainly be performed.

There is a great overlap in the mammographic and sonographic findings of benign and malignant breast lesions. For this reason many lesions that ultimately prove to be benign must be biopsied. When the radiologist recommends such a course for a suspicious occult lesion, the probability that the lesion will be malignant is about 25% to 30%. Each radiology practice calculates its own positive predictive value of mammography in lesions recommended for biopsy, but the range is generally 25% to 30%. Women who are anxious about undergoing biopsy should be told that the outcome is benign 70% to 75% of the time.

In a minority of cases the lesion visualized by mammography is so classically malignant that the diagnosis of cancer is virtually assured. Patients who receive such reports must be counseled to expect this diagnosis. Expeditious biopsy is extremely important for these women.

Biopsy

Biopsy is recommended in up to 3% of women undergoing screening mammography for the first time. There are several options available when biopsy of an occult lesion is recommended. The one most commonly used is the excisional biopsy preceded by a radiologic localization, however image-guided fine needle aspiration and needle core biopsy are quickly becoming alternatives in those communities in which resources for their performance are available.

Localization and Excisional Biopsy

Excisional biopsy of an occult breast lesion must be preceded by a localization. Because the lesion cannot be felt, the surgeon must have a guide to ensure that the mammographically visible abnormality is removed; the wire or dye inserted into the lesion by the radiologist provides this guidance. The majority of these lesions are benign so removal of the smallest piece of tissue possible is desirable for cosmetic reasons.

Localizations can be performed by inserting a wire into the lesion or by injecting blue dye (e.g., toluidine blue) into the area of the lesion. Placement of a wire is currently the favored technique because it allows more exact surgery. In either case a needle is placed through or adjacent to the lesion using mammographic guidance. The patient sits with her breast compressed in the mammography unit during this procedure. Although local anesthetic occasionally is used prior to needle placement, this is discouraged because it can obscure the lesion. Most localizations only require one needle stick. Ultrasound also is used sometimes to guide needle placement.

Once the needle is correctly positioned, a localizing wire or blue dye can be placed through it (Fig. 6-27). The woman then proceeds to the operating room where the surgeon uses the localization to guide excision of the occult lesion. After excision, the tissue should be taken to the radiology department for filming to be sure that the abnormality has been removed (Fig. 6-28). Following confirmation that the targeted abnormality has been removed, the tissue is transported to pathology.

Fine Needle Aspiration and Needle Core Biopsy

Fine needle aspiration (FNA) biopsy and needle core biopsy (NCB) also are performed to diagnose occult breast lesions. FNA is performed with a thin needle (usually 22 or 25 gauge) and yields a sample for cytologic analysis, whereas NCB is performed with a 14- or 15-gauge needle fired by a biopsy gun. NCB yields a sample of tissue that can be examined histologically so the special expertise of a cyto-

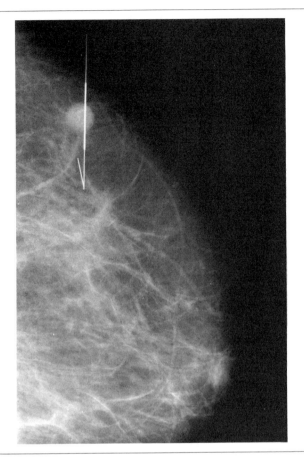

Fig. 6-27. Final film from a needle localization showing the hookwire passing through a well-circumscribed 1-cm mass that proved to be a metastasis from a renal cell carcinoma.

pathologist is not required. If the lesion can be visualized, both NCB and FNA can be performed using ultrasound guidance (Fig. 6-29).

Stereotaxic mammography units have also been developed to guide needle placement for percutaneous breast biopsies. In general stereotaxic NCB is performed on a dedicated unit, that is, a unit used only for that purpose. The patient lies prone on the x-ray table with her breast through the aperture (Fig. 6-30). Stereotaxic x-ray views are taken at +15- and −15-degree views with respect to a line that is perpendicular to the compression plate. The position of the lesion in each of these views is used to determine its three-dimensional location within the breast. The calculations of the coordinates are made by computer and the needle guide is then adjusted to these coordinates. The core needle is introduced and its prefire location at the proximal edge of the lesion is checked by film. After the needle

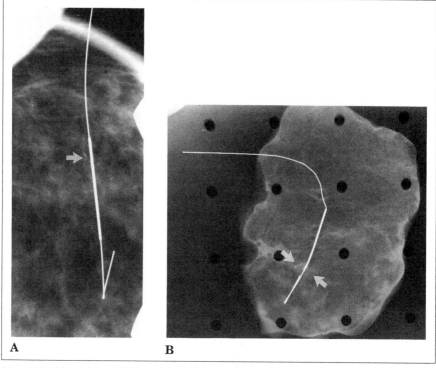

Fig. 6-28. Final film (A) from a needle localization of some suspicious microcalcifications *(arrow)*. The specimen radiograph (B) shows the calcifications *(arrows)* to be within the resected tissue. The diagnosis was comedo-type intraductal carcinoma.

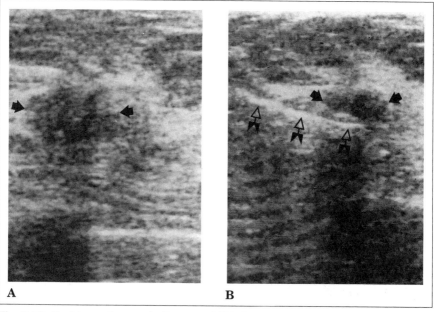

Fig. 6-29. Prebiopsy *(arrows)* ultrasound (A) shows a 1.4-cm solid mass *(arrows)* in the breast. Needle core biopsy was performed under ultrasound guidance (B). The 15-gauge core biopsy needle *(open arrows)* can be seen penetrating the mass *(filled arrows)*. The diagnosis was infiltrating ductal carcinoma.

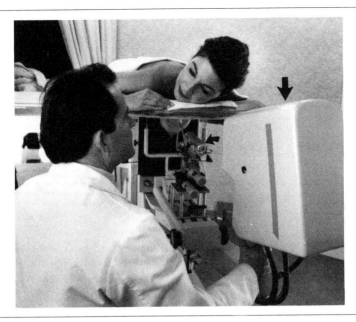

Fig. 6-30. Dedicated stereotaxic breast biopsy unit. The patient lies prone with her breast through the aperture in the table. The fenestrated compression paddle has been applied to the superior surface of the breast. The x-ray tube *(straight arrow)* can be rotated to take two views at +15 degrees and −15 degrees from a line perpendicular to the compression paddle. The location of the lesion in three dimensions can then be calculated and the needle guide *(curved arrow)* adjusted to the appropriate coordinates for accurate needle core biopsy. (Courtesy of Fischer Imaging Corp., Denver, CO.)

has been fired, its location is again checked to ensure that the lesion has been sampled. At least five core samples usually are obtained. Patients may develop some postprocedure bruising at the biopsy site. Other than one case of malignant seeding along the needle track, no significant complications from NCB have been reported.

Both FNA and NCB are far less expensive and less disfiguring than excisional biopsy. These procedures take about 1 hour to perform and women can return to their normal activities immediately afterward. In recent studies both FNA and NCB have shown accuracy rates similar to those of surgical biopsy. FNA, however, suffers from difficulty in obtaining adequate numbers of cells for diagnosis. When cancer is diagnosed by FNA, noninvasive lesions cannot be differentiated from those that are invasive.

Many studies are under way to further define the roles for FNA and NCB in the diagnosis of occult breast lesions. It is likely that NCB will become more widely used in the future. It appears to be a cost-effective alternative to surgical biopsy that, in many cases, can be performed with existing resources. Women who undergo FNA or NCB must, however, understand that the lesion has only been sampled—it has not been removed. They must be encouraged to return for regular follow-up according to the protocol established by the radiologist.

Clinicians should discuss the availability of the various methods of biopsy with the radiologists in their community.

Suggested Reading

Kopans DB, et al. Spring hookwire breast lesion localizer: Use with rigid-compression mammographic systems. *Radiology* 157:537, 1985.

Kopans DB. Standardized mammography reporting. *Radiol Clin North Am* 30:257, 1992.

Lindfors K. Breast Imaging. In WE Brant and CA Helms (eds). *Fundamentals of Diagnostic Radiology*. Baltimore: Williams & Wilkins, 1994.

Parker SH, Lovin JD, Jobe WE, et al. Nonpalpable breast lesions: Stereotactic automated large-core biopsies. *Radiology* 180:403, 1991.

Sickles EA. Mammographic features of 300 consecutive nonpalpable breast cancers. *AJR* 146:661, 1986.

Sickles EA. Practical solutions to common mammographic problems: Tailoring the examination. *AJR* 151:31, 1988.

Sickles EA. Periodic mammographic follow-up of probably benign lesions: Results in 3,184 consecutive cases. *Radiology* 179:463, 1991.

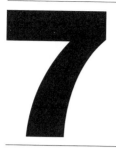

The Palpable Breast Mass

Lois F. O'Grady,
Karen K. Lindfors,
Lydia Pleotis Howell,
and Virginia Joyce

Discovery of a mass in the breast arouses anxiety in both patient and physician. Both are concerned about the possibility of cancer, and the practitioner knows, as well, that the second most common cause of legal actions against physicians is the failure to diagnose breast cancer. The approach to the patient with a palpable breast mass will vary, depending on her age and other aspects of her clinical history, such as pregnancy or lactation, previous surgeries, and previous diagnoses of benign breast changes or cancer. Careful physical examination is mandatory, and it is reviewed in detail in this chapter.

History

The history should include the customary information on how long the mass has been present, whether it changes in size with the menses, and how quickly it changes. In addition, the information listed in Table 7-1 should be obtained. A recent pregnancy with nursing might be associated with a galactocele. A coincident nipple discharge, especially from a single duct, would increase suspicion of malignancy. Hormonal therapy might increase nodularity. Trauma to the breast could produce hematoma, fat necrosis, or a ruptured cyst. History of a prior mass and its diagnosis is important: a prior biopsy showing severe hyperplasia or atypia raises a large red flag, but a biopsy showing a low-risk lesion should not provide a false sense of security. A personal or family history of breast cancer is critical, as is a history of any coincident major medical condition.

Table 7-1. Important findings from history in patient with palpable mass

Phase of menstrual cycle
Recent pregnancy or lactation
Nipple discharge
Hormone use
Trauma
Prior biopsy diagnosis
Cancer history
Other medical conditions

Physical Examination

A careful, thorough breast examination is mandatory and provides the opportunity to instruct each woman in a simple reproducible method of breast self-examination (see Appendix A). Ideally, the breast should be examined just after the menstrual cycle when it is less full and less tender. This may not be possible when evaluating a newly discovered mass. The room should be well lit, and the examination should begin with the patient sitting at ease with her arms at her side (Fig. 7-1B). Most women have breasts that are dissimilar in size but any exaggerated size differences may reflect underlying pathology. The breast contour is inspected for signs of dimpling or retraction. These same signs are sought while the patient changes position—holding her arms over her head and placing her hands on her hips while exerting pressure—to exaggerate subtle changes (Fig. 7-1C, D).

With the woman still sitting, the axillae should be palpated for enlarged, firm, or matted lymph nodes. Supporting the woman's elbow with one of the examiner's hands (Fig. 7-2A), or having her

Fig. 7-1. Examination of the breast—inspection. A. The lighting is poor, creating too many shadows on the breast. B, C, and D. More direct lighting and position changes permit better appreciation of subtle changes in contour.

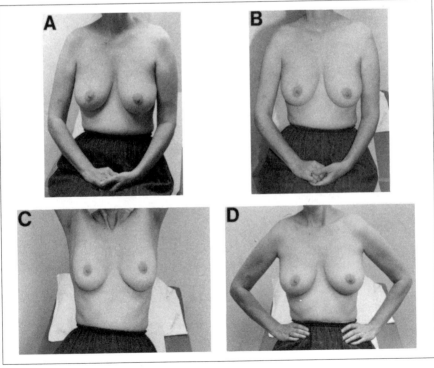

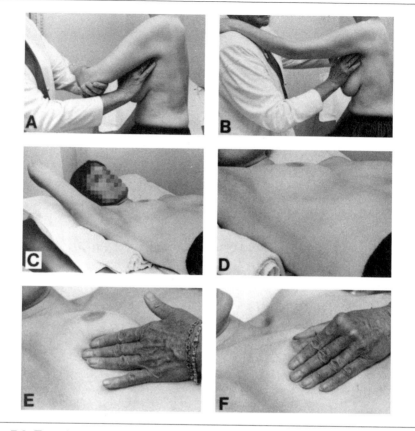

Fig. 7-2. Examination of the breast—palpation. A and B. Support of the patient's arm, by either technique, relaxes the shoulder muscles and permits deeper palpation of the axillae. C and D. Palpation of the breast is enhanced if the arm is placed over the head and the body is slightly hyperextended thus stretching the breast over the chest wall. E. Detection of irregularities and nodularity is enhanced if the flat surface of the fingers is used to palpate the breast tissue, using rotatory or linear motion to pass the breast tissue between the fingers and the chest wall. F. A nipple discharge can be elicited by using the hand to gently compress the breast tissue while the thumb and index finger gently squeeze the nipple-areolar complex.

rest her arm on the examiner's shoulder (Fig. 7-2B), facilitates deep palpation into the axillae.

Palpation of the breast is best accomplished with the patient supine. To examine the right breast, the patient's right arm is placed over her head, and a small pillow or folded towel may be placed under her shoulder (Fig. 7-2C). This stretches the breast across the chest wall (Fig. 7-2D) and facilitates palpation. The process is repeated for the opposite side. The breast is palpated with the flat portion of the examiner's fingers (Fig. 7-2E), and the breast tissue is passed between the fingers and the firm structures of the chest wall. This technique facilitates detection of nodularity and masses. The pattern used to cover the entire breast, from the clavicle to the inframammary fold and from the sternum to the midaxillary line, can be horizontal, circular, or vertical (see Appendix A). Each examiner, whether clinician or patient, should establish his or her own pattern so as to be consistent. The nipple should be gently squeezed to check for discharge (Fig. 7-2F). Many physicians use a breast diagram, similar to that seen in Appendix B, to record areas to be checked in future examinations.

If the patient has discovered an abnormality, the patient and physician should agree about the area in question.

Breast masses can be very subtle, even to the most astute examiner, and there are frequent questions about the significance of clinical findings. If there is any question as to whether a subtle mass or thickening requires investigation, reexamination 4 to 6 weeks later, in the midcycle of a premenopausal woman, is in the best interest of the patient and the practitioner. The appointment for reexamination should be clearly recorded.

None of us has a microscope in our fingertips, and only a tissue sample can make a firm diagnosis of a breast mass. There are a few points, however, that suggest (*suggest* only) that a mass may be benign or malignant (Table 7-2). Benign masses tend to be moveable, tend to have easily distinguished margins, and tend to feel like the rest of the breast. A mass of glandular tissue will often partially disperse into cords with gentle manipulation and is often mirrored on the opposite side. A multiplicity of masses also suggests a benign diagnosis.

Malignancies tend to be firm or hard and to have margins that are not quite clear. They feel different from the rest of the breast, do not disperse with palpation, and are not mirrored on the opposite side. Any mass that is fixed to the skin or chest wall should be considered malignant.

Diagnostic Evaluation of a Breast Mass

In Women Over Age 30

The first step in the diagnostic evaluation of a new mass in this age group is a mammogram. Although some authors suggest that needle aspiration is the first approach, we disagree. Even in the most expert hands, needles in breasts can produce hematomas that can obscure the mammographic interpretation of the suspicious area for several weeks.

There is a major caveat to remember in this discussion: *the most common mistake made is to assume that a "negative" mammogram means a nonmalignant mass. A "negative" mammogram indicates only that the radiologist sees no radiographic evidence of malignancy.* Eight to ten percent of cancers in this age group will not be seen on mammography, thus, a palpable mass must be investigated fully. A

Table 7-2. Important findings from examination in patient
with palpable mass

Suggests benign	Suggests malignant
Soft	Firm, hard
Discrete	Indistinct
Mobile	Fixed
Multiple	Solitary
	Nipple retraction
	Skin dimpling
	Bloody discharge

reasonable approach to the patient with a palpable mass is outlined
in Fig. 7-3.

In performing the mammogram, a radiopaque marker should be
placed on the patient's skin over the mass to assist the radiologist
in evaluating the specific area of concern. It will also ensure that
what is felt is the same as what is seen. Such correlation is important
in ensuring that a palpation-guided fine needle aspiration (FNA) or
biopsy will encompass the area of mammographic concern.

Fig. 7-3. Work-up of a palpable mass in women over age 30.

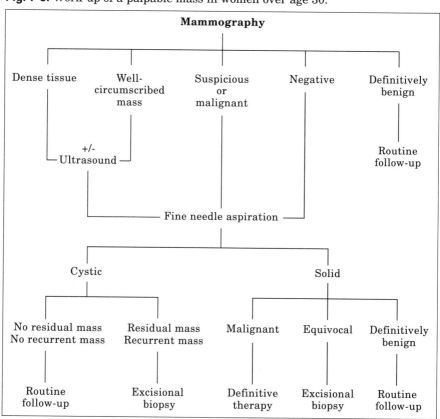

The primary reason for performing mammography in women with palpable masses is to assess the affected breast for multifocal cancer or more extensive subclinical disease, such as extensive intraductal cancer, which is especially important if breast-conserving therapy is contemplated (Fig. 7-4). The second reason is to examine the contralateral breast for suspicious abnormalities because the potential for bilateral breast cancer is well known. Mammography may also be helpful in definitively diagnosing the palpable abnormality as benign, thus avoiding a biopsy. Fat-containing masses (lipoma, oil cysts, lymph nodes, hamartomas, etc.) and densely calcified fibroadenomas are two types of lesions that can be confidently diagnosed as benign on mammography (Fig. 7-5).

Lesions that are not clearly benign mammographically must be evaluated further. Following mammography, FNA is recommended as the next step in diagnosis. It has been shown that when the cytologic results from FNA are combined with the mammographic and physical findings (triple test), over 95% of all breast cancers are detected, and the accuracy of benign diagnoses is equivalent to that of histologic examination. FNA has been found to be particularly useful in the evaluation of vague, nondiscrete thickenings because it is often difficult to identify a corresponding lesion on the mammogram. Surgery for diagnosis alone can thus be avoided in many

Fig. 7-4. Craniocaudal (A) and magnification compression (B) views of the right breast demonstrating multifocal infiltrating duct carcinoma. A palpable 2-cm mass *(straight arrows)* was located anterolateral to the 1-cm occult lesion *(curved arrows)*.

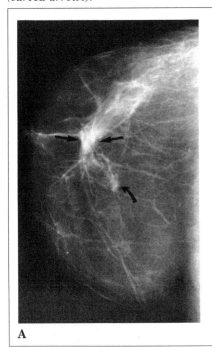
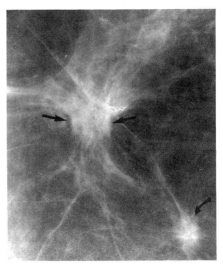

A   B

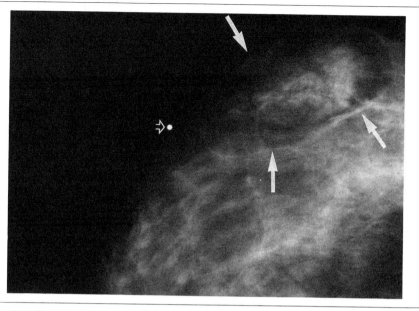

Fig. 7-5. Craniocaudal view of the right breast in a woman with a 4-cm mass on physical examination. A radiopaque marker *(open arrow)* was placed on the skin at the site of the palpable abnormality. This correlated with a benign fat-containing mass *(solid arrows)* on the mammogram. This is the typical appearance of a hamartoma (fibroadenolipoma), which is benign and does not require biopsy.

cases. Appropriate treatment can be tailored according to the cytologic diagnosis. Follow-up is essential.

Equivocal cytologic diagnoses must be followed by excisional biopsy and, of course, a malignant finding sets in motion a separate chain of events (see Chaps. 13, 14, and 15). Fortunately, in experienced laboratories, equivocal or suspicious cytologic diagnoses from breast FNAs are relatively uncommon. At our institution, only 4% of all breast aspirates are called suspicious and when they are excised most turn out to represent carcinoma. A suspicious diagnosis is therefore an important and meaningful diagnosis that must be pursued.

If mammography is negative in a patient with a clinically evident mass and dense breasts, ultrasound is often suggested as a subsequent imaging study to determine whether the mass is solid or a simple cyst. Ultrasound may also be suggested when a mass is shown to be round and well circumscribed and a cyst is suspected. Ultrasound can be diagnostic of simple cysts, which are never malignant. If, however, therapeutic aspiration is desired, FNA can be performed. After a cyst is drained, there should be no residual mass, and the cyst should not recur within 3 months. If there is a residual mass, or a recurrence, biopsy is suggested. If no fluid can be aspirated from the mass, it is presumed to be solid, and cells can be withdrawn for cytologic evaluation.

In Women Under Age 30

Figure 7-6 provides a guide for the diagnostic evaluation of a new palpable mass in women under the age of 30, when cancers are rare (but not unheard of), and the risk of mammography may be of some concern.

There is controversy regarding the efficacy of mammography in this particular age group. Some experts believe that there is a significant decrease in the sensitivity of this test, possibly due to the higher proportion of women with dense breasts. A recent study has shown that, overall, mammography can demonstrate 89% of cancers in women under 35 years of age. Even in women with very dense breasts, 75% of the lesions could be seen mammographically. The rationale for avoiding mammography in young women is based primarily on the possibility of increased risk of radiogenic breast cancer (see Chap. 4).

Initial evaluation of focal masses can be made with ultrasound or FNA. Although ultrasound can determine whether a mass represents a simple cyst, it cannot distinguish solid benign masses from malignant ones. For this determination FNA is required.

Because FNA is both diagnostic and therapeutic for cysts as well as highly specific in diagnosing solid masses, it is an excellent initial diagnostic method. As mentioned in Chap. 5, FNA is safe, easily performed in the office, highly accurate, and more cost-effective

Fig. 7-6. Work-up of a palpable mass in women under the age of 30.

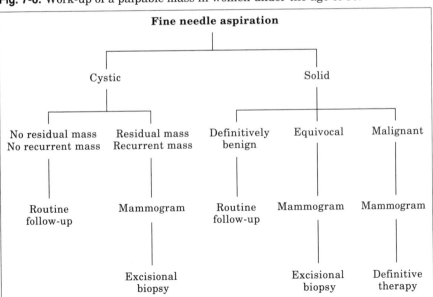

when compared to excisional biopsy. By actually sampling the lesion and examining it microscopically, FNA provides a confidence that clinical follow-up cannot.

If the FNA yields cystic fluid that does not appear bloody or necrotic, and there is no residual mass, either immediately after the aspiration or 3 months later, the patient may be reassured and returned to routine care. If there is a residual mass or the cyst continues to recur, mammography and surgical biopsy should be performed, as discussed above for older patients.

If the mass is solid, and the FNA shows a clearly and definitively benign condition (e.g., fibroadenoma), the patient may be returned to routine care. Many patients prefer to have fibroadenomas removed for aesthetic reasons. If the mass is not removed, any sudden change in size or texture should be brought to medical attention because fibroadenomas can harbor malignant transformation, albeit very rarely.

Equivocal findings from FNA (e.g., insufficient tissue, suspicious cytology, or lack of correlation with clinical findings) require excisional biopsy. Mammography should be performed before surgery. If cancer is found at the time of FNA, mammography can then be performed. The radiologist should be made aware that an aspiration has been performed. The intervention may confound mammographic assessment of the palpable area, because hematomas can look similar to carcinomas, but if carcinoma has already been diagnosed this is immaterial. The assessment of surrounding tissues and of the contralateral breast will not be compromised. Of course, a malignant pathology requires appropriate intervention. Carcinoma is extremely rare in women under 30 years of age. In one series of 542 surgical biopsies in women in this age group, cancer was found in only four cases (0.8%).

Biopsies that reveal florid hyperplasia, especially atypical hyperplasia, may alter the risk profile of the patient and call for closer supervision (see Chap. 12).

In Women with a History of Cancer

In patients who have had a lumpectomy or mastectomy for the treatment of breast cancer, local or regional recurrence is expected to occur in 10% of these patients and can be as high as 40% in patients with primary tumors that are either locally advanced or have extensive axillary involvement.

Mammography is less sensitive following breast conserving therapy (55–75%) because of the frequent scarring and radiation-induced changes that occur in the treated breast. Nevertheless, mammography is complementary to physical examination in the detection of a recurrence. Similar numbers of tumors will be discovered by both techniques, and each technique will miss a significant number of recurrences. Once again, it is important to stress that *especially in the treated breast* a negative mammogram should not deter performance of FNA of a clinically detected mass.

Nodules frequently occur near surgical scars, and it is difficult to evaluate clinically whether these represent suture granulomata, a remodeled scar, or a recurrent tumor. FNA is an easy and accurate method with which to evaluate these lesions. FNA of surgical scar lesions in women with breast cancer has shown a diagnostic accuracy of 98.2% and a sensitivity and specificity of 97.4% and 100%, respectively. The results are optimized when the FNA is performed by someone with experience, because the dense fibrosis that comprises a scar can "bind down" malignant cells, making them difficult to remove by aspiration.

If the patient has had reconstruction, the recurrent mass may be in the reconstructed breast. If the reconstruction has been done with implants placed under the pectoralis major muscle (preferred by oncologists), recurrent masses should be readily apparent and accessible for needle biopsy. Subglandular implants (i.e., anterior to the pectoralis major muscle) make mammography more difficult; to avoid rupturing an implant, needle biopsy may best be done under radiographic control. In these patients excisional biopsy may be preferred.

It should be noted that tissue reaction to the implant or its contents can produce masses of inflammatory or scar tissue.

Reconstruction using myocutaneous flaps is popular. Although there is no true breast tissue, recurrences can occur deep under the reconstruction and can create a mass effect. These are difficult to detect; if suspected, sophisticated radiologic imaging techniques may be required.

Diagnostic Evaluation of a Mass in Males

Men may develop gynecomastia from a number of causes (see Chap. 2). One-third may be unilateral, but even when bilateral, male gynecomastia is often asymmetric. Mammography is very helpful in differentiating gynecomastia from malignancy, as can be seen in Fig. 2-7.

Similar to its role in the evaluation of breast masses in women, FNA can play a similar role in the evaluation of masses in men. Gynecomastia has a distinctive cytomorphologic pattern and, in fact, can be distinguished from fibrocystic changes and fibroadenoma without knowledge of the patient's sex. Breast carcinomas in men are readily differentiated cytologically from gynecomastia and resemble those seen in women.

Thus the approach to the patient would include careful exclusion of the typical causes of gynecomastia, followed by mammography and FNA.

Suggested Reading

Medical Legal Issues

Kern KA. Causes of breast cancer malpractice litigation. *Arch Surg* 127:542–547, 1992.

Masses in Women Under 30

deParedes ES, Marsteller LP, and Eden BV. Breast cancers in women 35 years of age and younger: Mammographic findings. *Radiology* 177:117–119, 1990.

Ferguson CM, and Powell RW. Breast masses in young women. *Arch Surg* 124:1338–1341, 1989.

Gupta RK, Dowle CS, and Simpson JS. The value of needle aspiration cytology of the breast, with an emphasis on the diagnosis of breast disease in young women below the age of 30. *Acta Cytol* 34: 165–168, 1990.

Masses in Women Over 30

Butler JA, Vargas HI, Worthen N, and Wilson SE. Accuracy of combined clinical-mammographic-cytologic diagnosis of dominant breast masses: A prospective study. *Arch Surg* 125:893–896, 1990.

Donegan WL. Evaluation of a palpable breast mass. *N Engl J Med* 327:937–942, 1992.

Hermansen C, et al. Diagnostic reliability of combined physical examination, mammography, and fine-needle puncture ("Triple Test") in breast tumors. *Cancer* 60:1866–1871, 1987.

Kopans DB, et al. Palpable breast masses: The importance of preoperative mammography. *JAMA* 246:2819–2822, 1981.

Langmuir VK, Cramer SF, and Hood ME. Fine needle aspiration cytology in the management of palpable benign and malignant breast disease: Correlation with clinical and mammographic findings. *Acta Cytol* 33:93–98, 1989.

Masses in Women with a History of Cancer

Dershaw DD, McCormick B, Cox L, and Osborne MP. Differentiation of benign and malignant local tumor recurrence after lumpectomy. *AJR* 155:35–38, 1990.

Malaberger E, et al. Fine-needle aspiration and cytologic findings of surgical scar lesions in women with breast cancer. *Cancer* 69:148–152, 1992.

Orel SG, et al. Breast cancer recurrence after lumpectomy and irradiation: Role of mammography in detection. *Radiology* 183:201–206, 1992.

Masses in Men

Bhagat P, and Kline T. The male breast and malignant neoplasms. *Cancer* 65:2338–2341, 1990.

Kapdi CC, and Parekh NJ. The male breast. *Radiol Clin North Am* 21:137–148, 1983.

Russin VL, Lachowicz C, and Kline T. Male breast lesions: Gynecomastia and its distinction from carcinoma by aspiration biopsy cytology. *Diagn Cytopathol* 5:243–247, 1989.

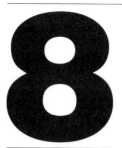

The Painful Breast

Lois F. O'Grady

A patient's complaint of breast pain can be caused by myriad disorders from actual breast disease to cardiac angina. To begin to identify the etiology of the discomfort, one must rely on the old standbys of medical care—a careful history and a careful physical examination.

The symptom of breast pain should be analyzed carefully in terms of whether it is cyclical or noncyclical. Cyclical pain is typical of fibrocystic disorders of the breast and noncyclical pain can be caused by breast disease or other (nonbreast) diseases (Table 8-1).

The physical manifestation of the pain can be analyzed by physical examination: Is there tenderness to palpation of the breast and chest wall? If so, is that tenderness in the breast itself or in the structures of the chest wall? There are several ways to determine this information. One is to ask the patient whether she perceives the discomfort when the breast or the chest wall is examined. Another is to examine the patient in both recumbent and leaning-forward positions. When the patient is recumbent, one is palpating the breast tissue by a rotatory motion of the fingers, allowing the breast tissue to pass between the fingers and the chest wall. Discomfort from this examination could be from the breast itself, or because the examiner is pressing on chest wall structures. Again, the patient's opinion should be sought. Next, the patient should sit up and lean forward so that the breast is falling away from the chest wall. In this position, it is possible to palpate the breast without touching the chest wall and to pass the examining fingers in back of the breast to palpate the chest wall. Using this technique, it is usually possible to identify the principal points of tenderness—breast, rib or overlying muscle, or joint (costrochondral). Again, the input of the patient is critical: Where does she perceive the discomfort during palpation of various areas, or is there any tenderness at all?

If the solution to the clinical problem is not evident on the initial physician-patient interaction, it is very helpful to have the patient keep a monthly calendar to daily record the presence or absence of her symptomatology and its relative severity ($+$ to $++++$). Over a 2-month course of time, the pattern is usually quite evident, and the focus of the clinical investigation can be directed accordingly.

Table 8-1. Cyclical versus noncyclical breast pain

Cyclical pain	Noncyclical pain
Fibrocystic disorders	Breast disorders
	Chest wall disorders
	Bone
	Muscle
	Joint
	Pleural disease
	Cardiac disease

Cyclical Breast Pain

The patient who has pain that cycles with the menstrual cycle, and which is localized to the breast, almost invariably has fibrocystic changes. The patient usually has lumpy breasts on palpation. The etiology of this condition is discussed in Chap. 2.

This chapter will review the therapy of the fibrocystic type of benign breast disease, which can be defined as the syndrome of mastalgia associated with varying degrees of lumpiness of the breast.

Etiology

Although the exact etiology of the fibrocystic component of benign breast disease may not be known, there can be no question that it is tied to cyclic hormonal stimulation. It begins after the menarche, cycles with the menses, and is worse just before menstruation. It worsens over time, and it goes away after menopause, whether that menopause is natural or induced. It can be made worse by exogenous estrogen, and it can be improved by any therapeutic maneuver that counteracts estrogen. It is presumed to result from excess estrogen, deficient progesterone (in the gynecologic literature it is referred to as the disease of the failed corpus luteum), or both. Some have suggested that individual variation, or regional tissue variation, in sensitivity to estrogen plays a role, but this has never been confirmed.

Therapy

Because many therapeutic interventions will interfere with physiologic function, a few basic tenets should be kept in mind:

1. Not all patients need therapy.
2. Try simple things first.
3. Interfere with physiologic function as little as possible.
4. Reserve the most onerous therapy for the patient with the most onerous disease.

5. Constantly check to be sure that the side effects of therapy are not worse than the disease (the old therapeutic index or risk/cost-benefit analysis).

Therapy can be divided into two major categories: nonhormonal and hormonal (Table 8-2). There is, in all probability, a significant placebo effect to all.

Nonhormonal Therapy

REASSURANCE. Patients with only mild premenstrual mastalgia may experience enough relief to learn that this is a physiologic phenomena and that no therapy is required.

SUPPORT. A properly fitting support brassiere, especially in women with large breasts, may provide relief by preventing some of the drag on the ligamentous support of the breast when the breasts are full and tense with fluid.

DIURESIS. Those patients who have significant swelling of the breast with each menstrual cycle (a change of one or two bra cup sizes), and who have a generalized tense, tight discomfort, may have significant relief from a diuretic given for 1 week prior to the menstrual period.

NSAIDs. Nonsteroidal antiinflammatory drugs, with or without diuretics, may add enough relief that other interventions are unnecessary.

WEIGHT LOSS. Steroid precursors can be converted to estrogen in fat tissue, and obese women have high endogenous estrogen levels. This is thought by many to be the underlying etiology in obese

Table 8-2. Relative value of treatment

Treatment	Probably effective	Probably worthless
Nonhormonal		
Reassurance	+	
Bra support	+	
Diuresis	+	
NSAIDs	+	
Weight loss		−
Caffeine abstention		−
Lipids		−
Vitamins		−
Hormonal		
Oral contraceptives	++	
Progesterone	+	
Androgens	+++	
Antiprolactin	++	
Antiestrogens	+++	
LH-RH agonists	too early to know	

NSAIDs = nonsteroidal antiinflammatory drugs; LH-RH = luteinizing hormone-releasing hormone; + = somewhat effective; ++ = effective; +++ = very effective; − = not effective.

women of increased risks of endometrial and breast cancer. If one believes that estrogen-progesterone imbalance is behind at least some benign breast disease, it follows that significant weight loss should help. It makes sense, is recommended by many (including me), but not all. It must be remembered that significant weight loss, increased well-being and activity may affect physiologic systems besides estrogen.

CAFFEINE ABSTENTION. In 1989, Minton updated his original work that suggested that methylxanthines (as found in coffee, tea, chocolate, etc.) alter cyclic adenosine monophosphate (AMP) metabolism and produce the fluid retention and the fibrous-glandular proliferation of fibrocystic disease. He now focuses less on caffeine and suggests that abnormal catecholamine metabolism is linked to the phenomenon. His view that complete abstention from caffeine will improve fibrocystic disease has become popular. Although some patients swear that it makes a difference, objective controlled trials show no benefit.

LIPIDS. Exactly how or why anyone ever tried it is not clear, but in 1981 an article in a prestigious journal by a distinguished group reported that oil from the evening primrose flower, ingested in capsule form, helped breast pain. As it turns out, evening primrose oil has a very high content of essential fatty acids (with 72% linoleic acid) and is claimed to favorably influence prostaglandin metabolism, an abnormality of which is claimed to cause fibrocystic disease. This group, from Cardiff, Wales, has recently backed down a little on their favor for this oil. Regardless, the Cardiff group has done more work than many in this area of breast disease, their influence is strong, and the oil will probably be recommended by them for some time. The oil has very few side effects, which is why it may be favored by patients and physicians.

VITAMINS. At various times vitamin E, pyridoxine, niacin, and other vitamins have been claimed to be of benefit, but no valid claim exists for any of them.

Hormonal Therapy

Aimed at counteracting the effect of estrogen or prolactin, a variety of regimens have evolved, as summarized in Table 8-3. Table 8-4 compares the cost of various hormonal therapies.

ORAL CONTRACEPTIVES. In 1978, it was noted that users of oral contraceptives had less fibrocystic disease. This finding has been amply confirmed and reconfirmed. The protective effect appears to be the result of the exogenous progesterone. If oral contraceptives could prevent fibrocystic disease, the next logical step was to try them as therapy. Indeed, they work very well for a large percentage of patients with moderate mastalgia. The current recommendation is to use the newer, low estrogen/high progesterone combinations (0.02-mg ethinyl estradiol and 1-mg norethindrone acetate), which are reported to provide an 88% response rate.

Table 8-3. Hormonal therapies

	Dose	Side effects
Oral contraceptive	0.02-mg ethinyl estradiol 1-mg norethindrone	Well tolerated
Progesterone	10-mg PO medroxyprogesterone acetate, days 15–25 of menstrual cycle	Fairly tolerated, some weight gain
Danazol	200–400 mg PO daily for 2–3 months, then 100 mg/day for 2–3 months	Amenorrhea, weight gain, masculinization at higher dose
Bromocriptine	2.5 mg, PO, bid for 3 months	Poorly tolerated, nausea, dizziness, hypotension, fertility problems
Tamoxifen	10 mg, PO, once or twice a day	Well tolerated, hot flashes, amenorrhea at high doses
LH-RH agonists	1 mg subcutaneous monthly	Full range of menopausal symptoms

Table 8-4. Cost comparison of hormonal therapies

Drug	Regimen	Cost*
Oral contraceptive	0.02-mg ethinyl estradiol 1-mg norethindrone 3 monthly cycles	$60
Progesterone	10-mg PO medroxyprogesterone acetate, days 15–25 of menstrual cycle 3 monthly cycles	$19
Danazol	200 mg/day PO for 3 months 400 mg/day PO (2 × 200 mg/day) 100 mg/day PO (2 × 50 mg/day)	$200 $400 $160
Bromocriptine	2.5 mg PO bid for 3 months	$200
Tamoxifen	10 mg PO bid for 3 months	$231
Zolodex (LH-RH analog)	3.6-mg implant monthly × 3	$1000

*In 1992 wholesale dollars, for 3 months of therapy.

Oral contraceptives are familiar drugs to the patient and the physician. They cause few side effects. Their favorable therapeutic ratio is well known, although the therapeutic effect takes time to occur—4 to 6 months—which is a relative disadvantage. Also, the disorder worsens within months of stopping the oral contraceptives. At one time there was concern that the use of oral contraceptives in women over age 35, the age at which fibrocystic disease becomes prevalent, was questionable because of an increased risk of thromboembolic disease. However, the low estrogen preparations are reasonably safe, particularly in women who do not smoke. The patient must, of course, be told of any possible risk and, together with the physician, must decide whether the degree of breast discomfort is worth the risk.

PROGESTERONE. While the effects of the oral contraceptives were being documented in Britain and the United States, workers in France, led by Maurvais-Jarvis, were documenting that many women with fibrocystic breast disease had lower-than-average levels of progesterone during the last half of their menstrual period. Their finding that the corpus luteum secreted less progesterone in these women led to a popular concept in the gynecological literature—that fibrocystic disease was a disease of the "failed corpus luteum." The therapeutic use of progesterone has proved effective.

Medroxyprogesterone, 10 mg, PO, days 15 to 25 of the monthly cycle, is preferred in the United States, but other schedules (lower daily dose) work as well. Percutaneous (topical) administration of progesterone is common in Europe. Fifty mg of progesterone in a cream base is massaged into each breast, and about 10% of the dose is absorbed.

The drug is more effective than oral contraceptives for patients with more severe disease, and its effect is seen sooner, often within the first month. The side effects are weight gain and some adverse effect on lipid metabolism, which are of concern if the drug is to be used for years rather than months, or if seen in patients who already have lipid abnormalities or cardiovascular disease. Some patients on the higher doses complain of a "fuzzy" feeling in the head, a decreased ability to concentrate and analyze, a sense of unsteadiness or instability of gait, and significant mood changes. These disappear within days of discontinuing the drug. Again, the patient and physician must weigh benefit versus cost.

ANDROGENS. If the therapeutic goal is to counteract the effect of estrogen, androgen is an effective means of achieving this goal. *Danazol,* an androgen variant, reduces levels of follicle-stimulating hormone and luteinizing hormone, with concomitant decreases in estrogen. Because it is a variant androgen, its masculinizing properties, although present, are not prominent.

Several dosage regimens for danazol have been proposed. The most commonly recommended dosage is 200 to 400 mg per day for 4 to 6 months, but others have shown that lower doses can be effective, with fewer side effects. Once a remission is attained, it can last for several months after the drug is discontinued. If it recurs, lower doses may maintain a remission after it is reinduced.

Danazol is a powerful drug. It induces remissions quickly. Patients note symptomatic relief within a week or two, and after a few months of therapy, there is objective, mammographically documented clearing of the disease and a decrease in the size of cysts. Powerful drugs tend to have powerful *side effects* and danazol is no exception. Amenorrhea occurs in 50% of patients (it is dose related and reversible);

headaches, hot flashes, and irritability can occur; and the androgenic effects of weight gain, oily skin, acne, and hirsutism are seen with higher doses. Obviously, the drug, in full dosage, should be reserved for the most severe cases. The number of women willing to take the drug and put up with the side effects is mute testimony to the severity of the symptoms in some.

ANTIPROLACTIN. Some Italian physicians have long held the view that prolactin, rather than excess estrogen, is the cause of fibrocystic disease. Prolactin levels have never been shown to be elevated consistently in fibrocystic disease, and attention has now turned to abnormalities of chronobiologic rhythmic prolactin release as etiologic factors. Despite this, *bromocriptine,* a long-acting dopaminergic drug that inhibits prolactin release, has been reported consistently to produce improvement in fibrocystic disease, both subjectively and objectively. The drug is given as 2.5 mg twice a day for several months.

Bromocriptine is another powerful drug and has major *side effects* including nausea, vomiting, postural hypotension, and dizziness. Even ardent supporters of the drug report that 20% of patients drop out from studies because of intolerance. It also must be remembered that this drug has major effects on fertility. It is used in Europe, but is not widely used by American physicians.

ANTIESTROGENS. If a therapeutic goal is to counteract the effect of estrogen, what better way than with an antiestrogen drug? *Tamoxifen,* widely used in the adjuvant therapy of breast cancer, blocks estrogen receptors. In doses of 10 mg, once or twice a day for 3 months, it is very effective, subjectively and objectively, in treating fibrocystic disease. Over 70% of patients respond. Like androgen, the drug quickly induces responses that last for several months after the drug is discontinued. Lower dose maintenance may be effective for recurrent disease.

There are *side effects*. Amenorrhea at the higher doses is most common. The drug shares with oral contraceptives a slightly increased risk of thromboembolic disease (under 1%), but it has nowhere near the side effects of bromocriptine or danazol. Its longterm use (months) has been associated with mild vaginitis and endometrial hyperplasia but these would not be of concern with short courses of therapy. There is now convincing evidence available that long-term use of the drug has a favorable effect on bone density, serum lipid profile, and cardiovascular disease (see Chap. 15). And yet, the drug has not yet "caught on," perhaps because of its association with the treatment of malignant disease.

Now that the tamoxifen breast cancer prevention trials are under way and the long-term safety of the drug has been established, perhaps the medical community will use it more. It is safer and better tolerated than bromocriptine or danazol. It should not take much more favorable evidence for it to be the primary drug for therapy.

Table 8-5. Recommendations for treatment*

Mild to moderate symptoms	Moderate to severe symptoms
1. Try nonhormonal maneuvers for 3 months. If no relief:	1. Progesterone for 2 to 3 months. If no relief:
2. Oral contraceptives for 3 months. If no relief:	2. Tamoxifen, 10 mg bid. If no relief:
3. Progesterone for 3 months. If no relief:	3. Danazol, 400–600 mg/day
4. Tamoxifen	

*Not recommended: Bromocriptine and LH-RH agonists (outside a clinical trial).

LUTEINIZING HORMONE-RELEASING HORMONE (**LH-RH**) **AGONISTS.** In the past few years drugs have become available that act as agonists to gonadotropin-releasing hormones. After initial stimulation and release of hormones, there is effective blockade. The potent antigonadal action of LH-RH agonists induces complete ovarian inhibition, which results in low levels of estradiol, progesterone, ovarian androgens, and prolactin. In an excellent initial study that includes hormone receptor analysis of biopsy specimens and radiologic examinations, the drug shows great promise. It has the advantage of being formulated for monthly subcutaneous injections, however, it may prove to have many side effects. Clinical trials are needed before it can be recommended for routine use.

Surgical Management
There are rare patients in whom fibrocystic disease is debilitating and in whom drugs either do not work or are not tolerated. There is one drastic option: mastectomy with reconstruction. It is not recommended lightly and only after significant soul searching and consultation.

Summary

In summary, the fibrocystic component of benign breast disease is probably caused by real or relative hyperestrinism. Therapies, hormonal and nonhormonal, are available that can improve the disease in a large number of patients. Table 8-5 summarizes the author's recommendations for treatment.

Noncyclical Breast Pain

Differential Diagnosis

The differential diagnosis for patients with noncyclical breast pain is presented in Table 8-6.

Table 8-6. Differential diagnosis for noncyclical breast pain

Hematoma (posttraumatic)
Fat necrosis
Ruptured cyst
Infection
Tumor

Hematoma

The breast is an exposed organ, subject to trauma day in and day out. Occasionally the trauma is enough to produce a bruise or hematoma that can cause discomfort for several days. Usually the history will suffice to make this diagnosis.

Fat Necrosis

Fat necrosis can occur spontaneously or as the result of trauma. It produces localized areas of tenderness and sometimes swelling. Fat necrosis can be difficult to distinguish from cancer because they often look the same on mammography. The symptoms, however, usually abate in about a month, whereas the signs and symptoms of cancer persist. Often, the diagnosis is made at biopsy.

Ruptured Cyst

If a patient with known cystic disease experiences trauma to the breast (e.g., nonpenetrating injury, steering wheel or seat belt trauma from a car accident, or compression for a mammogram) a cyst may rupture. The onset of symptoms is usually sudden and associated with the physical event. The cyst's contents induce an inflammatory reaction that causes the symptoms. As with fat necrosis, the symptoms and signs of swelling and tenderness experienced with a ruptured cyst disappear over the course of a month. This is one of the reasons we emphasize that breast disorders can be watched for a month (no more) before definitive investigations are begun.

Infection

Infection in the breast is usually evident, with signs of redness, swelling, and tenderness. Antibiotics are the obvious therapy. The usual infecting organisms are skin flora, thus the antibiotics chosen should be specific for gram-positive organisms, as, for example, the semisynthetic penicillins. Small areas of infection can be treated with oral antibiotics, but extensive infection may require intravenous therapy for a day or two. Abscesses or extensive infection may need surgical treatment.

A major clinical point to be made is that infections are common in lactating breasts but in the absence of distinct reasons for the infection, for example, bites (human or insect) or penetrating trauma, infections are very rare in nonlactating breasts. A 7- to 10-day course of antibiotics is appropriate, but *if the infection does not clear readily, steps should be taken to ensure that the infection is not inflammatory cancer.* Incision, drainage, and biopsy will be required after general evaluation similar to that done for a palpable mass (see Chap. 7). It must be recognized, however, that the patient's discomfort may preclude a mammogram or that interpretation of the mammogram may be difficult due to changes produced by the infection.

Tumor

Tumors are a rare cause of breast discomfort. Most present as painless masses. But they present with discomfort often enough that if a cause for breast discomfort is not evident, a mammogram is warranted to exclude underlying pathology. (One must always remember that mammograms are not infallible and have a 10% margin of error.) Mammographic abnormalities or masses detected on physical examination should be evaluated by biopsy.

Noncyclical Pain Not Localized to the Breast

Differential Diagnosis

The differential diagnosis of this type of chest discomfort can be a challenge to even the most astute diagnostician (Table 8-7).

Chest Wall

Any disorder of the chest wall structures can produce pain that can be interpreted as being of breast origin. Fractures of the ribs often, but not always, have a history of trauma. Rib fractures caused by radionecrosis of bone (after radiation therapy to the breast or chest wall) may occur spontaneously or with minimal trauma. And certainly tumors metastatic to the ribs can lead to pain. Physical examination which suggests that the pain is localized to the bony struc-

Table 8-7. Differential diagnosis of noncyclical pain not in the breast

Chest wall
  Bone disease
  Fracture
  Tumor
Muscle
  Fibromyositis
Joint
  Costochondritis
Pleura
  Infarct
  Embolus
  Sickle cell disease
  Tumor
  Infection
Heart
  Angina

tures can be investigated by nuclear scans or radiographic procedures. If these are positive, bony origin of the pain is confirmed.

Muscle

Fibromyositis, a variant collagen vascular disease, involves the chest
wall and often the structures of the shoulder and back as well. Localized areas of thickening and tenderness in the muscle bodies and
relief of symptoms by antiinflammatory drugs confirm the clinical
diagnosis.

Joint

Costochondritis presents with tenderness in the costochondral junc-
tions, accompanied by local swelling. It is usually evident on examination. Exacerbation with motion and relief with antiinflammatory
drugs confirm the clinical impression.

Pleura

Any disease of the pleura, whether an infarct from embolus, pneu-
monic processes, or irritation by tumor can produce chest wall pain
and tenderness to palpation. Its noncyclical nature, without any
obvious chest wall pathology, leads one to radiographic examination
of the chest, which provides evidence of the underlying pathology.

Heart

A rare bird, perhaps, but more than one female patient with typical
or atypical angina has ended up visiting a physician interested in
breast disease. The illogic assumption that women do not have ischemic cardiac disease is well entrenched in the mind set of clinicians.
The clues to appropriate diagnosis are the relation of the pain to
exercise or stress; confirmation is with appropriate cardiologic investigation (ECG, treadmill, or thallium scans).

Suggested Reading

General

Brinton LA, et al. Risk factors for benign breast disease. *Am J Epidemiol* 113:203–214, 1981.

Dannerstein L, et al. Progesterone and the premenstrual syndrome:
A double blind crossover trial. *Br Med J* 290:1617–1621, 1985.

Drukker BH, and deMendonca WL. Fibrocystic change and fibrocystic disease of the breast. *Obstet Gynecol Clin North Am* 14:685–702,
1987.

Fornander T, et al. Long-term adjuvant tamoxifen in early breast
cancer: Effect on bone mineral density in post menopausal women.
J Clin Oncol 8:1019–1024, 1990.

Hughes LE, Mansel RE, and Webster DJT, (eds). *Benign Disorders and Diseases of the Breast*. London: Bailliere-Tindall, 1989.

Love RR, et al. Effects of tamoxifen therapy on lipid and lipoprotein levels in post menopausal patients with node negative breast cancer. *J Natl Cancer Inst* 82:1327–1332, 1990.

Maddox PR, and Mansel RE. Management of breast pain and nodularity. *World J Surg* 13:699–705, 1989.

Minton JP, and Huss AI. Nonendocrine theories of the etiology of benign breast disease. *World J Surg* 13:680–684, 1989.

Sismondi P, et al. Benign breast disease, an update. *Clin Exp Obstet Gynecol* 17(2):57–116, 1990.

Sitruk-Ware LR, et al. Inadequate corpus luteal function in women with benign breast disease. *J Clin Endocrinol Metab* 44:771–774, 1977.

Vorherr H. Fibrocystic breast disease: Pathophysiology, pathomorphology, clinical picture, and management. *Am J Obstet Gynecol* 154: 161–179, 1986.

Drug Therapy

Colin R, Gaspard V, and Lambotte R. Relationship of mastodynia with its endocrine environment and treatment in a double blind trial with lynestrenol. *Arch Gynak* 225:7–13, 1978.

Dogliotti L, and Mansel RE. Bromocriptine treatment of cyclical mastalgia/fibrocystic breast disease: Update on European trial. *Br J Clin Pract Symp Suppl* 68:26–32, 1992.

Fentiman IS, et al. Double-blind controlled trial of tamoxifen therapy for mastalgia. *Lancet* 1:287–288, 1986.

Fentiman IS, et al. Dosage and duration of tamoxifen treatment for mastalgia: A controlled trial. *Br J Surg* 75:845–846, 1988.

Maddox PR, Harrison BJ, and Mansel RE. Low dose danazol for mastalgia. *Br J Clin Pract Symp Suppl* 68:43–47, 1989.

Monsonego J, et al. Fibrocystic disease of the breast in premenopausal women: Histo-hormonal correlation and response to luteinizing hormone releasing hormone analog treatment. *Am J Obstet Gynecol* 164:1181–1189, 1991.

Parazzini F, et al. Methylxanthine, alcohol-free diet and fibrocystic disease: A factorial clinical trial. *Surgery* 99:576–578, 1986.

Tobiassen T, et al. Danazol treatment of severely symptomatic fibrocystic disease and long term follow-up—The Hjorring project. *Acta Obstet Gynecol Scand Suppl* 123:159–176, 1984.

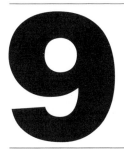

Nipple Discharge

Lois F. O'Grady,
Karen K. Lindfors,
Lydia Pleotis Howell,
and Virginia Joyce

The breast exhibits some secretory activity throughout most of adult life. The difference between lactating and nonlactating breasts is chiefly in the degree of secretion, and to a lesser degree in the chemical composition of the fluid. In nonlactating women, the nipple ducts are occluded by keratin plugs, thus, secretory material does not ordinarily appear on the nipple, but is instead degraded within the ducts and then resorbed. How long it remains in the ducts is not known.

Nipple discharge is the third most common breast condition for which women seek medical attention, following closely behind lumps and mastalgia. As more women perform breast self-examination, more discover the discharge. In fact, fluid can be expressed from the breast in 50% to 60% of Caucasian and African-American women, and in about 40% of Asian-American women.

There is increasing interest in the significance of breast secretions and their relation to breast disease. Endogenous and exogenous hormones are secreted into the ducts along with potential carcinogens that women may acquire from their diet or environment. Some women may secrete more actively than others, and major differences may exist in the length of time that the secretions remain in contact with the duct epithelium.

Character and Significance of the Discharge

There is consensus among breast disease experts that fluid appearing only with manipulation of the breast and nipple is rarely associated with pathology and merely reflects normal physiology. Nipple discharges that may be of concern are those that

1. truly come from the nipple ducts,
2. appear spontaneously,
3. are persistent, and
4. are nonlactational.

Although some experts try to separate the discharges into multiple categories based on color and consistency, the majority seem to fall into three types as shown in Table 9-1. Of these, only those that appear serous or bloody are associated with underlying malignancy with any degree of frequency. They can be considered together.

Types of Nipple Discharge

Table 9-2 provides a guide for the differential diagnosis of a nipple discharge considered to be significant. The most common type of discharge is a *milky discharge* (cloudy, whitish or almost clear color, thin, nonsticky). It can be physiologic, that is, resulting from lactational events or from increased mechanical stimulation of the nipple from suckling, fondling, or irritation by clothing during prolonged repetitive exercise (e.g., jogging). Both male and female adolescents may experience a milky discharge during puberty. Drugs that stimulate prolactin secretion, have estrogenic properties, or affect the hypothalamic-pituitary axis can cause galactorrhea (see Chap. 2). Excess prolactin either from the pituitary or from ectopic causes can do the same. Because all of these conditions affect both breasts, this discharge is likely to be bilateral and from multiple ducts. Regardless of the cause, a milky discharge does not result from intrinsic breast disease. If it is copious, an endocrine evaluation should be done.

The second most common type of nipple discharge is an *opalescent discharge*. Thicker than a milky discharge, it may be somewhat sticky or gummy and may vary in color from creamy to yellow to

Table 9-1. Types of nipple discharge

Type of discharge	Typical color
Milky	Whitish or almost clear
Opalescent	Clear to yellow, green, brown, or black
Bloody or serous	Red, pink, or brown (rarely, clear/watery)

Table 9-2. Causes of major types of nipple discharge

Milky	Opalescent	Serous or bloody
Physiologic	Duct ectasia	Pregnancy
Mechanical stimulation	Cyst	Duct ectasia
Postlactational		Hyperplastic duct lesions
Drugs		Papilloma
Prolactin		Papillomatosis
Phenothiazine		Cancer
Reserpine		
Estrogenic		
Opiates		
Pathologic		
Hypophyseal/pituitary		
tumors		
Ectopic prolactin		
(bronchogenic cancer)		

green to brown or black. If it is brown or black, a standard chemical test (e.g., Hematest) will confirm the absence of blood. Opalescent discharge usually results from ectasia in one or multiple ducts or from drainage from cystic dilatations of ducts deeper in the breast in which normal secretions have collected and partially decomposed. It may be unilateral or bilateral and usually (but not always) involves multiple ducts. Again, it is rarely associated with malignant disease of the breast. If it is from multiple ducts, it needs no investigation or treatment unless the amount of discharge is socially embarrassing to the patient.

The third type, which is the least common type, is that of the *serous, serosanguineous, or frankly bloody nipple discharge.* A clear watery discharge has been associated with the same types of disorders, but it is very rare. It is in this group that there is some chance of finding significant underlying pathology. Even so, blood is produced most commonly by benign disorders. Duct ectasia can produce enough local inflammation to cause bleeding, and there are reports of sanguineous discharge beginning in the second trimester of pregnancy when the breast tissue proliferates rapidly and some of the benign duct lining becomes necrotic. It is benign. The discharge from ectasia or pregnancy is more likely to be bilateral and from more than one duct, whereas the discharge caused by cancer or papilloma is almost always unilateral and reproducibly secreted from one duct.

Even in patients with worrisome discharges (serous, bloody, and perhaps clear watery), cancer is the cause in only 10% to 15%. In one series of patients undergoing surgery for suspicious discharges (Table 9-3) the most common finding was a papilloma. Cancer was present in only 11% and the remainder were due to benign conditions. In another series of 259 breast biopsies performed to investigate nipple discharge, only half of those found to have cancer had a bloody discharge, and slightly more than half of the papillomas presented with bloody discharge. Of note is that about one-sixth of the patients in this series who had duct ectasia had a bloody discharge. It appears, therefore, that although a serous or bloody discharge can be associated with cancer or papilloma, cancers and papillomas can induce nonbloody discharges. Conversely, bloody discharge is often due to benign conditions.

Table 9-3. Etiology of suspicious nipple discharge in a group of surgical patients

Etiology	Percentage
Papilloma/papillomatosis	44
Duct ectasia	23
Fibrocystic disease	16
Cancer	11

Approach to the Patient with Nipple Discharge

Evaluation

After a detailed history with attention to reproductive status and drug history is taken, a careful physical examination is in order. The patient should in a recumbent position with her ipsilateral arm raised over her head to stretch the breast over the chest wall. The breast should be compressed with both hands in a "milking" motion to see if fluid can be expressed. Careful notation should be made of the color and consistency of the fluid, whether it is unilateral or bilateral, and whether it comes from one or multiple ducts on the nipple. If no secretion appears, ask the patient to express the fluid.

If the discharge is unilateral and comes from one or two ducts, the breast should be carefully stroked or milked with one finger in that particular quadrant to see if a point can be found that triggers the discharge. This point should be carefully noted for the surgeon. Next, the breast should be carefully examined for a dominant mass, with particular attention given periareolar and infraareolar areas. If a mass is found, it must be investigated as such. The investigation of the palpable mass (see Chap. 7) should not be delayed and takes priority over concern for the discharge.

In the absence of a palpable mass, patients may be separated by the character of the fluid to assist in establishing a diagnosis. Although much work has been done on the analysis of breast fluid, there is so much inconsistency in the findings and such a high false-negative rate for underlying malignancy that routine chemical or pathologic analysis of the fluid is not recommended. Cytologic evaluation is an inefficient method with low sensitivity and is reliable only if frankly positive, which occurs in less than 1% of patients. In a mass screening study in Japan, 20,537 nipple discharges were examined cytologically and only 18 cancers and 61 papillomas were detected. It has been suggested that only bloody discharges be examined cytologically. If the physician elects to do this, care should be taken to collect the first drop of fluid expressed because it will contain the most exfoliated cells that have pooled in the duct and thus will have maximum cellularity for cytologic diagnosis.

If the discharge is purulent and if the areolar complex shows signs of inflammation, cultures should be obtained and appropriate antibiotic treatment given (including antistaphylococcal coverage). Once the infection has resolved, the patient should be observed carefully for 3 to 4 months to be sure that there is no recurrence or underlying disease.

Management

Using the information gathered from the history and physical examination, one can proceed as indicated in Fig. 9-1.

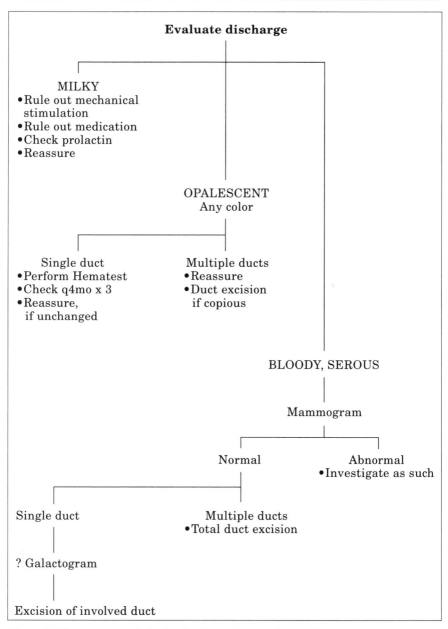

Fig. 9-1. Management of nipple discharge in a patient without a mass.

Milky discharge is not associated with breast pathology and as long as the serum prolactin is normal (no pituitary or other tumor), the patient may be reassured.

Patients with opalescent discharge may be separated according to whether the discharge is from a single duct or multiple ducts. The patient may be assured that the latter is always benign. One may take this opportunity to instruct the patient in breast self-examination and to order routine screening mammography if it is appropriate to her age. No investigation is necessary, but if the quantity of the discharge causes social embarrassment, excision of the ductal complex may be done. These patients are usually beyond the typical child-bearing age so the ability to nurse is not of major significance, but the patients should be warned that ductal excision may well interfere with nipple sensation.

Opalescent discharge from a single duct may be more suspicious. If the color is anything other than creamy white, Hematest of the fluid is advised to make sure that it is not sanguineous. If no blood is found, there is no mass, and if the mammogram is negative the patient may be watched and no intervention is needed at this time.

A serous, sanguineous or a clear, watery discharge requires careful evaluation. In patients with pathologic discharge mammography should be performed first. The mammograms may show the etiology of the discharge. Ductal carcinoma in situ may be seen as malignant microcalcifications. Some solitary papillomas can be visualized mammographically as soft tissue masses. However, most frequently the mammograms are negative in otherwise asymptomatic patients.

An abnormality found on mammogram must be investigated as such and takes precedence over investigation of the nipple discharge.

If the mammogram is normal, the patients may be subdivided according to whether the discharge is from multiple ducts or from a single duct. If from multiple ducts, it is extremely unlikely to be malignant. If the discharge stains clothing and causes embarrassment or undue concern, a major duct excision may be performed with the understanding that subsequent nursing is not possible and that there will be altered nipple sensation.

A serous or bloody discharge from a single duct is the most worrisome condition of all. It *must* be investigated carefully. The next step, however, is controversial. Consultation with the surgeon is helpful in deciding whether galactography will be necessary or useful. Some surgeons prefer to cannulate the involved duct in the operating room and to dissect along the cannula. Some inject blue dye into the duct to guide the dissection. Others prefer that galactography be done to localize the suspected lesion preoperatively, as demonstrated in Fig. 9-2.

Galactography is performed in the radiology suite. It is contraindicated in patients with active mastitis. It is important that the discharge be expressible on the day of the procedure so that the radiologist can identify the duct of concern. Patients should be advised against nipple manipulation for a few days before the procedure. At the time of the procedure, the discharge is expressed and the duct to be cannulated is identified. A small blunt needle is inserted into the duct and contrast is injected. When the patient feels pressure, tightness, or pain, the injection is stopped and mammographic evaluation is done. The films are examined for evidence of intraductal masses. Benign lesions such as papillomas cannot be dis-

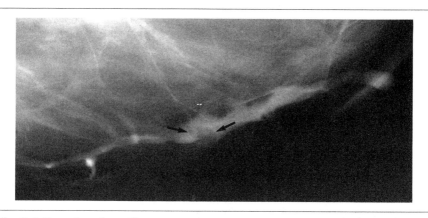

Fig. 9-2. Intraductal papilloma on galactography. The galactogram shows a lobulated intraductal mass *(arrows)* that proved to be an intraductal papilloma in this patient with a unilateral, spontaneous bloody nipple discharge. (Courtesy of Dr. Walter Tim, Lodi, California.)

tinguished from carcinoma, and a negative study does not guarantee the absence of pathology.

Some surgeons require a second galactogram on the day of surgery to reidentify the lesion. To facilitate dissection of the duct, this can be done in conjunction with injection of blue dye. Other surgeons prefer a needle localization of the intraductal abnormality.

A critical point, and one subject to discussion, is what to do in the face of a normal ductogram in a patient with a serous or bloody nipple discharge. Most agree that the duct must be excised. If this is to be done anyway, why bother with the ductogram in the first place? This excellent question is the primary reason why many surgeons do not request the test.

Duct excision is the treatment of choice. Whether the offending duct is identified by injection of methylene blue, or by painting the nipple with collodion for several days to allow the duct to distend, is the surgeon's choice. The procedure is usually done through a small curvilinear incision along the areolar border. In the absence of a gross abnormality, the duct is excised from its interface with the nipple to the place where it leaves the ductal complex and enters the breast parenchyma. It is not uncommon for the pathology to be so microscopic that it is not visible to the naked eye. The procedure is an outpatient one performed under local anesthesia. Nursing ability and nipple sensation are preserved. Further therapy will be required only if a malignancy is found.

In summary, the majority of nipple discharges are associated with nonmalignant changes in the breast. Those characteristics of nipple discharge that are more often associated with underlying malignancy are shown in Table 9-4. When these are present, careful investigation is warranted.

Table 9-4. Characteristics of nipple discharge associated with cancer

Spontaneous
Serous or bloody
Unilateral
Single duct
Associated with mass
Patient over age 50

Nipple Discharge in Males

At puberty gynecomastia is not uncommon and occasionally there is associated nipple secretion. Although it is of no medical consequence, it may be a significant social problem. Fortunately, it will cease within a few months. In adults, prolactin-secreting tumors and the same drugs that cause gynecomastia can lead to nipple discharge.

In general, however, nipple discharge in the adult male is more often associated with underlying malignancy than in the female. Mammography is mandatory, and biopsy should be done at the slightest hint of a mass or mammographic abnormality.

Suggested Reading

General

Carpenter R, Adamson A, and Royle GT. A prospective study of nipple discharge. *Br J Clin Pract Symp Suppl* 68:54–57, 1989.

Hughes LE, Mansel RE, and Webster DJT. *Benign Disorders and Diseases of the Breast.* London: Bailliere-Tindall, 1989. Pp 133–142.

Keynes G. Chronic mastitis. *Br J Surg* 11:89–121, 1923.

Leis HP. Management of nipple discharge. *World J Surg* 13:736–742, 1989.

Petrakis NL. Studies on the epidemiology and natural history of benign breast disease and breast cancer using nipple aspirate fluid. *Cancer Epidemiol Biomarkers Prev* 2:3–10, 1993.

Cytology

Ciatto J, Bravetti P, and Cariaggi P. Significance of nipple discharge clinical patterns in selection of cases for cytologic exam. *Acta Cytol* 30:17–20, 1986.

Johnson TL, and Kini SR. Cytologic and clinicopathologic features of abnormal nipple secretions: 225 cases. *Diagn Cytopathol* 7:17–22, 1991.

Takeda T, et al. Nipple discharge in mass screening for breast cancer. *Acta Cytol* 34:161–164, 1990.

Radiology

Fajardo LL, Jackson VP, and Hunter TB. Interventional procedures in diseases of the breast: Needle biopsy, pneumocystography and galactography. *AJR* 158:1231–1238, 1992.

Tabar L, Dean PB, and Pentek Z. Galactography: The diagnostic procedure of choice for nipple discharge. *AJR* 149:31–38, 1983.

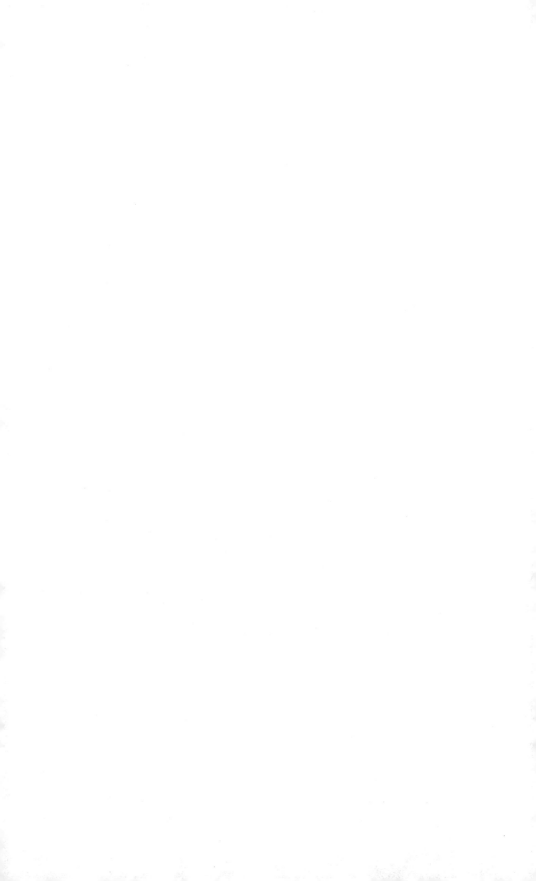

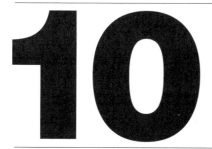

Estrogen Replacement Therapy

Richard H. Oi

The Benefits of Estrogen Replacement Therapy

There is substantial evidence to suggest that postmenopausal estrogen replacement therapy (ERT) is effective in ameliorating symptoms of vasomotor instability and genitourinary atrophy. More important, ERT protects against coronary artery disease and osteoporosis. Heart disease is the leading cause of death in postmenopausal women. Although there has not yet been a randomized controlled study, available epidemiologic data suggest very strongly that ERT has an independent and major protective effect against coronary heart disease. This protective effect is achieved by improving the lipoprotein profile, decreasing low-density lipoprotein (LDL) cholesterol, and increasing high-density lipoprotein (HDL) cholesterol; there also may be direct positive effects on the coronary arteries and other vessels. The reduction in heart disease risk is calculated to be between 30% and 70%, even in the presence of established risk factors. Even more conclusive documentation exists showing that ERT prevents, or at least delays, bone loss when taken immediately after menopause, and that long-term use reduces by 50% the risk of osteoporotic fractures, especially hip fractures with its attendant mortality and high morbidity and disability.

Estrogen replacement therapy therefore contributes to increased life expectancy by reducing deaths from osteoporotic fractures as well as from coronary artery disease. These significant benefits make estrogen replacement a consideration for all women who have demonstrated cessation of ovarian function, either naturally at menopause or surgically prior to the menopause.

Breast Cancer Risk

Despite the potential benefits of ERT, there is concern about the role of estrogens in breast cancer. Breast cancer is the most frequently diagnosed cancer in women and is second only to lung cancer as a cause of cancer death. Risk factors for breast cancer identify an estrogen-related association and include low parity, early menarche and late menopause, anovulation, obesity, and first childbirth after age

30. Indeed, there is substantial research literature, both epidemiologic and clinical, that links estrogens to breast cancer. Although data from innumerable epidemiologic studies on breast cancer risk have been inconsistent, there does appear to be an emerging consensus that ERT does not increase the risk of developing breast cancer, certainly not for women who have used estrogen for less than 5 years or who have used conjugated estrogens at doses of 0.625 mg or less. It may not be unreasonable therefore, to conclude that the use of ERT is associated with an unlikely but still unknown risk of developing breast cancer and that overall there is no statistical evidence of increased breast cancer risk with the use of postmenopausal estrogen therapy.

Type of Estrogen

The type of estrogen used in replacement therapy has some biologic significance. Although serum concentrations of estrone and estradiol are similar for daily oral administration of estradiol valerate or conjugated equine estrogen, pharmacokinetic and physiologic effects may differ depending on the type of estrogen used. Ethinyl estradiol is more potent than conjugated estrogens and has been associated with a 20% increase in breast cancer risk that increases with the length of exposure. It is probable that conjugated estrogens do not significantly increase risk and that there is no association with length of exposure. Overall, risks seem to be slightly higher in European studies in which synthetic estrogens are used as compared to studies from the United States, in which the predominant estrogens prescribed are conjugated estrogens.

Route of Administration

Most of the data are derived from studies of patients on oral estrogen and do not include transdermal use, which has had limited clinical experience thus far. Estradiol by injection has been associated with a fourfold elevation in breast cancer risk, indicating that parenteral administration may influence risk.

Dose

The dose of estrogen necessary to prevent bone loss (and probably for cardiovascular protection) is 0.625 mg of conjugated estrogen per day. Higher doses may influence the incidence of breast cancer. Several studies have identified that women who took greater than 0.625 mg/day of conjugated estrogen had an increased risk of breast cancer but that the 0.625-mg dose did not appreciably increase breast cancer risk. Similarly, the relative risk is also low with the 1.25-mg dose. Again, the data are inconsistent but suggest that doses greater than

0.625 mg are not necessary and, indeed, larger doses may increase the risk of thrombosis.

Duration of Use

Data on breast cancer cover a period of no more than 10 years and little information exists on long-term use. In considering the recommendation that women take estrogens for as long as 20 to 25 years, especially for osteoporosis protection, duration of use becomes an issue and has been considered a possible factor in breast cancer risk. The literature does not permit a definitive conclusion. Using 0.625-mg conjugated estrogen, an analysis by the Centers for Disease Control finds no convincing evidence of a positive relationship between duration of therapy and breast cancer risk. This study calculates that risk did not appear to increase until after at least 5 years of estrogen use and that after 15 years of use there was a 30% increase in risk. The group did include, however, premenopausal women or women who had used estradiol, which was associated with a relative risk of 2.2 after 15 years. Other reports have found a nonsignificant trend between duration of hormone replacement use and breast cancer risk or little change in risk with increasing duration of use.

Progestogen with Estrogen

Addition of progestogen (also called progestin) is necessary for patients on ERT because unopposed estrogen increases the risk of developing endometrial adenocarcinoma. Progestogen may attenuate the positive lipid profile that is seen with estrogen therapy but the type, dose, and schedule of administration commonly prescribed does not negate the positive changes. Progestogen does not attenuate the effect on bone mineral density and is effective in preventing bone loss.

Epidemiologic studies on the use of progestogen have been inconclusive; progestogen has been associated with increased as well as decreased breast cancer risk. In culture, progestogen inhibits the stimulatory effect of estrogen on human mammary cancer cells. Laboratory evidence suggests that the addition of some type of progestogen might counteract the mitogenic effect of estrogen on breast tissue, perhaps reducing breast cancer risk by regulating autocrine and paracrine growth factor secretion. One of the newer contraceptive progestogens, *gestodene,* because of its high affinity for receptor sites in breast cancer cells, has been demonstrated to arrest growth of human mammary cancer cells in culture, presumably by stimulating secretion of tumor growth factor (TGF) beta, a growth factor known to arrest growth of breast cancer cells. Lynestrenol, another contraceptive progestogen, given in contraceptive doses, was shown to demonstrate a 22% regression in 65 postmenopausal women with advanced breast cancer. Overall, however, there is no convincing evidence that progestogens either reduce or increase breast cancer risk.

Family History

A positive family history includes at least one first-degree relative with breast cancer. Some studies report an increased risk of breast cancer for women with a positive family history; these women with a positive family history had a significantly higher risk if they had ever used estrogen. Other studies, however, do not show this association, and report no link between family history and estrogen therapy and breast cancer risk. High estrogen doses and a positive family history may contribute to risk, but there is no unequivocal link between a family history of breast cancer and an increased risk with ERT. Thus, a positive family history for breast cancer would not be a contraindication to the use of ERT but would require the dedicated surveillance required for all patients on estrogen.

Benign Breast Disease

A history of benign breast disease does not contraindicate use of ERT. There are reports of lower observed breast cancer risk in women with atypical ductal hyperplasia and decreased risk in patients with histologic evidence of proliferative disease that was not influenced by ERT. Many other studies report that estrogen did not affect benign breast disease and did not appear to increase the risk of breast cancer.

Previous Breast Cancer

The risk of inducing a recurrence or otherwise influencing prognosis with estrogen use in patients previously treated for breast cancer is unknown. Estrogen replacement therapy may stimulate recurrence of micrometastases that may not appear until a later time and therefore may result in a shortened survival interval or ERT may promote the growth of a second primary malignancy because patients with breast cancer are at higher risk for a second malignancy. There are no data on long-term estrogen use in women with breast cancer. A clinical trial using 0.625 mg of conjugated estrogen and 0.15-mg norgestrel daily for a total of 6 months has been reported. Treatment was for hot flashes and urogenital atrophy, and all patients were followed for at least 2 years. Symptoms were relieved and there was no evidence of tumor reactivation. There may be a role, therefore, for short-term ERT to relieve vasomotor symptoms, which are often self-limited, and to relieve symptoms of urogenital atrophy, but long-term therapy, which appears to be necessary for cardiovascular and bone loss protection, is a separate issue. Patients with breast cancer retain a significantly elevated risk of death from this disease for up to 40 years after the original diagnosis. Absence of recurrence or new disease after 2 years of estrogen replacement does not give assurance that long-term use, necessary for cardiovascular and bone loss protection, is without risk.

In the 1990s there has been a significant shift toward earlier diagnosis of breast cancer. More women are diagnosed with in situ carcinomas with a 98% to 99% cure rate. With invasive cancers that are less than 2 cm in size, an 80% cure rate is reported. The majority of women with in situ carcinomas can expect to live an additional 30 to 40 years, and given the benefits of ERT in cardiovascular protection and prevention of osteoporosis, it may no longer be appropriate to deny these patients replacement therapy. A careful risk-benefit assessment can be made for each individual patient by looking at her chance of surviving 30 years (see Chap. 12), at her family history of cardiovascular disease, and at her female family history of osteoporosis. These survival assessments, however, are based on patients who have not had prior ERT. In a patient previously treated for breast cancer, there is no information as to whether long-term ERT will or will not increase the risk of recurrence or promote the appearance of a second breast malignancy. In patients with in situ carcinoma, the benefits of ERT probably outweigh the risks.

Estrogen Replacement Schedules

If, after careful consideration, the patient elects to use ERT, replacement can be prescribed as described in Tables 10-1, 10-2, and 10-3.

For patients with stage I breast cancer, short-term use of estrogen to relieve vasomotor symptoms or symptoms of urogenital atrophy is a reasonable consideration. Doses as low as 0.300 mg daily will obviate vasomotor symptoms. Treatment can be continued for 6

Table 10-1. Estrogen replacement schedule for continuous estrogen and cyclic progestogen

Oral estrogen	Transdermal estrogen
Conjugated estrogen[a] (Premarin), 0.625 mg daily Medroxyprogesterone acetate[b] (Provera), 10 mg per day, cyclically, first to thirteenth days of the month	Estradiol (Estraderm), 0.050-mg patch, placed Sunday and Thursday Medroxyprogesterone acetate (Provera), 10 mg per day PO, first to thirteenth days of month

[a]Conjugated estrogen 0.625 mg, or its equivalent dose such as transdermal estrogen, 0.050 mg, is the minimum dose necessary for bone loss prevention and cardiovascular protection.
[b]Medroxyprogesterone acetate (MPA), 10 mg daily for 13 days, is used to attenuate the proliferative effect of estrogen on the endometrium. Lesser doses for a shorter duration may be used, especially in thin women, but 10 mg for 13 days is the optimum schedule for almost all women. Withdrawal bleeding should occur after the MPA dose is completed. The endometrium should be sampled for hyperplasia if bleeding occurs other than at the expected time (after MPA administration is completed).

Table 10-2. Estrogen replacement schedule for continuous estrogen combined with continuous progestogen

Higher progestogen dose[a]	Lower progestogen dose[b]
Conjugated estrogen (Premarin) 0.625 mg PO daily	Conjugated estrogen (Premarin) 0.625 mg PO daily
Medroxyprogesterone acetate (Provera) 5 mg PO daily	Medroxyprogesterone acetate (Provera) 2.5 mg PO daily

[a]Women who are heavier, with more fat stores, should probably be placed on the 5-mg dose of medroxyprogesterone acetate (MPA) because progestogens are cleared more efficiently in fatty tissues. Irregular bleeding or spotting will occur for up to 6 to 9 months before patients become amenorrheic.
[b]The MPA dose can be reduced to 2.5 mg after amenorrhea is achieved. The endometrium should be sampled for hyperplasia if bleeding or spotting continues after 6 months and at anytime that bleeding occurs after the patient has become amenorrheic.

Table 10-3. Estrogen replacement schedule for vaginal estrogen[a]

Preparations[b]
Conjugated estrogen cream (Premarin vaginal cream), 0.625 mg per gm; 1 or 2 gm per day
Estradiol vaginal cream (Estrace), 1-mg estradiol-17β per gm; 2 to 4 gm per day
Dienestrol vaginal cream (Ortho Dienestrol Cream), 0.01%; 1 applicatorful daily

[a]Vaginal estrogens are absorbed readily and progestogen therapy is necessary with long-term use to protect the endometrium. Likewise, bleeding from the endometrium may occur and should be managed as it would be with oral or transdermal therapy.
[b]Apply cream intravaginally daily at bedtime for 3 weeks after which, with relief of symptoms, the cream can be applied 2 or 3 times a week to maintain a symptom-free state.

months or so and then discontinued to see if the vascular instability, which is often self-limited, has dissipated, at which time estrogen can be discontinued. Similarly, estrogens can be used to relieve genitourinary atrophy symptoms, either orally or with intravaginal estrogen creams, which can then be used on an as needed basis after initial therapy has effected symptomatic improvement. Long-term therapy should be offered only after a thorough discussion and clear understanding of the risks and benefits as described above. Other measures, such as exercise, dietary modifications, and pharmacologic agents other than estrogens, may be better methods to prevent bone loss and cardiovascular disease in some patients. These alternative measures need to be taken into consideration.

Summary

Despite extensive literature on the subject, the use of ERT is still associated with an unknown risk of breast cancer. Almost all epidemiologic studies indicate that ERT reduces the risk of ischemic heart disease and prevents bone loss, two important causes of morbidity and mortality among menopausal women. There is still resistance on the part of many physicians to embrace the unrestricted use of ERT because those studies reporting minimal to no risk of developing breast cancer with ERT are based on data that are, for the most part, observational. Two large randomized and controlled studies are now in place that address the question of overall risk of ERT as measured against the benefits. These are the ongoing Postmenopausal Estrogen/Progestin Intervention (PEPI) study and the Women's Health Initiative study of the National Institutes of Health. The former should report data within the next few years but the latter is a 13-year study that began in 1993.

Present data indicate that the risk of developing breast cancer from ERT is minimal. Because the potential of reducing cardiovascular deaths and the morbidity and mortality of osteoporosis is so substantial ERT should be offered to all women who are menopausal in an effort to significantly improve their quality of life and their life expectancy. Concerns about breast cancer should no longer be an impediment to prescribing estrogen at menopause because the overall benefit of estrogen replacement appears to outweigh the risk of developing breast cancer.

Estrogen replacement therapy in women who have had breast cancer is another issue. Short-term use in the management of early and intermediate symptoms of estrogen deficiency seems reasonable. The long-term use that is necessary for osteoporosis protection and probably for cardiovascular protection, however, presents a circumstance that is more difficult to justify given the unknown risk of promoting recurrences and enhancing the appearance of a second malignancy—events that would adversely affect the patient's prognosis and length of survival.

Suggested Reading

Breast Cancer Risk

Armstrong BK. Oestrogen therapy after the menopause—Boon or bane? *Med J Aust* 148:213–214, 1988.

Bergkvist L, et al. The risk of breast cancer after estrogen and estrogen-progestin replacement. *N Engl J Med* 321:293–297, 1989.

Colditz GA, Egan KM, and Stampfer MJ. Hormone replacement therapy and risk of breast cancer: Results from epidemiologic studies. *Am J Obstet Gynecol* 168:1473–1480, 1993.

Colditz GA, et al. Prospective study of estrogen replacement therapy and risk of breast cancer in postmenopausal women. *JAMA* 264: 2648, 1990.

Dupont WD, and Page DL. Menopausal estrogen replacement therapy and breast cancer. *Arch Int Med* 151:67–72, 1991.

Hunt K, et al. Long-term surveillance of mortality and cancer incidence in women receiving hormone replacement therapy. *Br J Obstet Gynaecol* 94:620–635, 1987.

Sillero-Arenas M, et al. Menopausal hormone replacement therapy and breast cancer: A meta-analysis. *Obstet Gynecol* 79:286–294, 1992.

Steinberg KK, et al. A meta-analysis of the effect of estrogen replacement on the risk of breast cancer. *JAMA* 265:1985–1990, 1991.

Thomas DB. Do hormones cause breast cancer? *Cancer* 53:595–604, 1984.

Cardiovascular Protection

Barrett-Connor E, and Bush TL. Estrogen and coronary heart disease in women. *JAMA* 265:1861–1867, 1991.

Sitruk-Ware R, and Ibarra de Palacios P. Oestrogen replacement therapy and cardiovascular disease in post-menopausal women: A review. *Maturitas* 11:259–274, 1989.

Stampfer MJ, et al. A prospective study of postmenopausal estrogen therapy and cardiovascular diseases: Ten-year follow-up from the Nurses' Health Study. *N Engl J Med* 325:756, 1991.

Tepper R, et al. Hormonal replacement therapy in postmenopausal women and cardiovascular disease: An overview. *Obstet Gynecol Surv* 47:426–431, 1992.

Wolf PH, et al. Reduction of cardiovascular disease-related mortality among postmenopausal women who use hormones: Evidence from a national cohort. *Am J Obstet Gynecol* 164:489–494, 1991.

Osteoporosis Protection

Ettinger B, Genant HK, and Cann CE. Long-term estrogen replacement therapy prevents bone loss and fractures. *Ann Intern Med* 102:319–324, 1985.

Genant HK, Baylink DJ, and Gallagher JC. Estrogens in the prevention of osteoporosis in postmenopausal women. *Am J Obstet Gynecol* 161:1842–1846, 1989.

Quigley MET, et al. Estrogen therapy arrests bone loss in elderly women. *Am J Obstet Gynecol* 156:1516–1523, 1987.

Riggs BL, and Melton LJ. Involutional osteoporosis. *N Engl J Med* 314:1676–1686, 1986.

Weiss NS, et al. Decreased risk of fractures of the hip and lower forearm with postmenopausal use of estrogen. *N Engl J Med* 303: 1195–1198, 1980.

Type of Estrogen and Route of Administration

Hammond CB, and Maxson WS. Estrogen replacement therapy. *Clin Obstet Gynecol* 29:407–430, 1986.

Hulka BS. Hormone-replacement therapy and the risk of breast cancer. *Cancer* 40:289–296, 1990.

Wren BG, Brown LB, and Routledge JDA. Differential clinical response to oestrogens after menopause. *Med J Aust* 2:329–332, 1982.

Dose and Duration of Therapy

Brinton LA, et al. Menopausal estrogen use and the risk of breast cancer. *Cancer* 47:2517–2522, 1981.

Hoover R, et al. Menopausal estrogens and breast cancer. *N Engl J Med* 295:401–405, 1976.

Lufkin EG, et al. Estrogen replacement therapy: Current recommendations. *Mayo Clin Proc* 27:201–223, 1988.

Ross RK, et al. A case control study of menopausal estrogen therapy and breast cancer. *JAMA* 243:1635–1639, 1980.

Progestogen and Breast Cancer

Anderson TJ, Ferguson DJP, and Raab GM. Cell turnover in the resting human breast: Influence of parity, contraceptive pill, age and laterality. *Br J Cancer* 46:376–382, 1982.

Baum M. Studies point to pill hope in breast cancer. *Hosp Doctor* 22: 36, 1989.

Ewertz M. Influence of noncontraceptive exogenous and endogenous sex hormones on breast cancer risk in Denmark. *Int J Cancer* 42: 832–838, 1988.

Gambrell RD Jr, Baier RC, and Sanders BI. Decreased incidence of breast cancer in postmenopausal estrogen-progestogen users. *Obstet Gynecol* 62:435–443, 1983.

Henderson BE, et al. Re-evaluating the role of progestogen therapy after the menopause. *Fertil Steril* 49(suppl):9S–15S, 1988.

Lippman ME, et al. Autocrine and paracrine growth regulation of human breast cancer. *Breast Cancer Res Treat* 7:59–70, 1986.

Nachtigall LE, et al. Estrogen replacement therapy II: A prospective study in the relationship to carcinoma and cardiovascular and metabolic problems. *Obstet Gynecol* 54:74–79, 1979.

Stoll BA. Effect of lyndiol, an oral contraceptive on breast cancer. *Br Med J* 1:150–153, 1967.

Benign Breast Disease and Cancer

Black MM, et al. Association of atypical characteristics of benign breast lesions with subsequent risk of breast cancer. *Cancer* 29:338–343, 1972.

Dupont WD, and Page DL. Risk factors for breast cancer in women with proliferative breast disease. *N Engl J Med* 312:146–151, 1985.

Dupont WD, et al. Influence of exogenous estrogens, proliferative breast disease and other variables on breast cancer risk. *Cancer* 63:948–957, 1989.

Eskin BA. Malignant potential of benign breast lesions: Implications for estrogen therapy. *JAMA* 266:1146, 1991.

Page DL, et al. Atypical hyperplastic lesions of the female breast. *Cancer* 55:2698–2708, 1985.

Estrogen Use After Breast Cancer

Bergkvist L, et al. The risk of breast cancer after estrogen and estrogen-progestin replacement therapy. *Am J Epidemiol* 130:221–228, 1989.

Brinkley D, and Haybittle JL. Long-term survival of women with breast cancer. *Lancet* 1:1118, 1984.

Brinton LA, Hoover R, and Fraumeni JF, Jr. Menopausal oestrogens and breast cancer risk: An expanded case-control study. *Br J Cancer* 54:825–832, 1986.

Carbone PP, and Dreicer R. Estrogen use after breast cancer. *JAMA* 261:3616, 1989.

Hibberd AK, Horwood LJ, and Wells JE. Long term prognosis of women with breast cancer in New Zealand: Study of survival to 30 years. *Br Med J* 286:1777–1779, 1983.

Stoll BA. Hormone replacement therapy in women treated for breast cancer. *Eur J Cancer Clin Oncol* 25:1908–1913, 1989.

Stoll BA, and Parbhoo S. Treatment of menopausal symptoms in breast cancer patients. *Lancet* 1:1278–1279, 1988.

Wile AG, and DiSaia PJ. Hormones and breast cancer. *Am J Surg* 157:438–442, 1989.

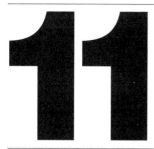

The Aesthetically Altered Breast

Debra A. Reilly
and Karen K. Lindfors

Over two million women in the United States have undergone contour-altering surgery of their breasts for aesthetic reasons. The most commonly performed procedures are augmentation, mastopexy, and reduction mammaplasty, in that order. The visible shape and form of the breasts, their radiographic appearance, and sometimes their function are altered by these techniques.

Breast Augmentation

Women who seek breast enhancement usually do so for the perceived problem of hypomastia (Fig. 11-1), for correction of an alteration in breast shape that has occurred with aging, or for correction of a mild or marked asymmetry of the breasts. Despite recent controversy concerning the use of silicone-based implants, many women are still seeking surgical consultation for augmentation. The actual number of women having augmentation surgery, however, has decreased by about 50% since 1991. For some women, breast enlargement surgery remains the only option for their goal of increasing self-esteem.

Implant Devices

In the early 1960s implants were introduced as an augmentation alternative to the injection of free silicone into the breasts. The implants were designed to resemble the shape of a young breast and were filled with a silicone gel that would mimic the texture of the breast parenchyma when placed under native tissue. Early implants included a single-lumen silicone bag or a shell filled with silicone gel; many manufacturers placed Dacron patches on the posterior surface of the implant to prevent migration. Later improvements in implant technology included (1) softening the texture of the shell and (2) removing the patches and adding a second outer lumen (thus the double-lumen implant) into which a variable amount of saline, antibiotics, or steroids could be placed. The surgeon could then tailor the procedure and create better breast symmetry. In the 1980s the smooth outer shell of the implant was replaced by some manufacturers with a textured surface, with the hope that this would reduce the incidence of capsular contracture around the implant.

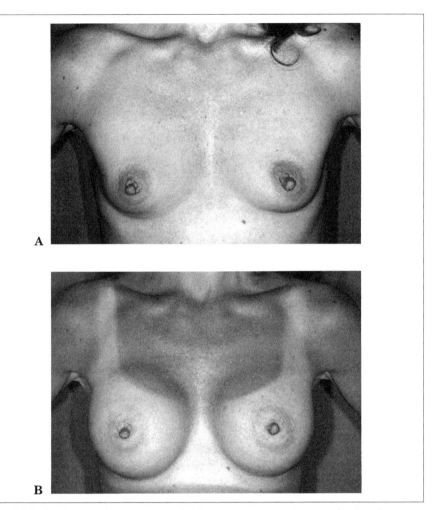

Fig. 11-1. A. Preoperative patient with hypomastia seen in consultation for an augmentation mammaplasty. B. The same woman 1 year after subglandular placement of silicone gel implants.

Saline-filled implants (Fig. 11-2) have also been used for breast augmentation, but it is commonly believed that silicone gel provides a consistency that more closely resembles that of native breast tissue. Silicone gel implants may also be superior in retaining their shape over time and in providing an acceptable contour despite changes related to pregnancy or aging. Some women have reported increased sensitivity to temperature extremes (especially colder temperatures) when saline-filled implants have been used (Table 11-1).

The Silicone Gel Controversy

Early in 1992, the United States Food and Drug Administration (FDA) imposed a moratorium on the use of silicone gel-containing

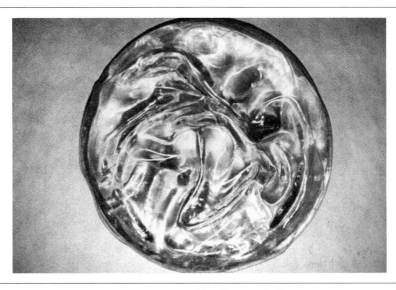

Fig. 11-2. Saline-filled breast implant with silicone shell.

Table 11-1. Silicone-filled versus saline-filled implants

	Silicone	Saline
Advantages	Natural feel Retains size and shape if intracapsular rupture	Readily available

Disadvantages	Gel bleed
	Questionable link with
	  systemic diseases
	FDA approved only for
	  reconstruction
		Cold hypersensitivity
		Rapid deflation with
		  rupture

implants for breast augmentation. These implants had initially been approved and released for insertion prior to legislation that now requires new devices to have premarket approval. The FDA is now requesting that the manufacturers present data in support of the implants, as if they were a newly developed product.

Concerns have been raised about possible manufacturing defects or implant misuse that could lead to implant rupture and leakage of the silicone gel. Silicone gel, once free in the tissue, may be taken up by macrophages and lymphatics and may "migrate" to adjacent soft tissue planes and lymph nodes. Occasional silicone particles have been found in nonadjacent organs, but because there are no unique markers for implant silicone their origin has not been definitely traced to breast implants.

The question has arisen as to whether leakage of silicone gel is linked to immune-related disorders and other systemic illnesses.

Symptoms reported by women with breast implants include pain (in the breast or generalized), fatigue, myalgias, arthralgias, rheumatoid problems, hair loss, memory loss, and neurologic disorders. To date there is no scientific evidence to support a causal relationship between silicone breast implants and any disease. Published epidemiologic studies have failed to find an association between breast implants and connective tissue disorders.

It has been theorized that silicone may induce a nonspecific immune response in women with sensitive immune systems. Unfortunately no serum assay for implant silicone is yet available, but research to develop such an assay is under way. Additional work has focused on identifying genotypes that may indicate increased sensitivity to silicone exposure.

Silicone gel-containing implants are now available only for women undergoing reconstructive breast surgery (e.g., postablative surgery for cancer, infection, trauma). This is done as part of a research protocol sponsored by the implant manufacturer and overseen by the FDA. Both the patient and the surgeon must sign the appropriate waivers and consent forms.

Saline-Filled Implants

Current technology allows surgeons to utilize saline-containing implants in women desiring augmentation. These are available as single or double lumens and come in a variety of shapes and sizes, with smooth or textured surfaces. The shape of the implants may vary from round to eccentric, and they may be stacked (with a larger implant against the chest wall and a smaller implant closer to the skin surface). All these variations are offered so that the surgical procedure can be tailored to best meet the patient's expectations.

It must be remembered that saline implants are surrounded by a silicone-containing bag or shell and that the potential local or systemic effects from this form of silicone are also unknown. The FDA is studying the safety and efficacy of these implants as well as implants containing other substances (i.e., peanut oil).

Benefit Versus Risk

Potential benefits of the use of implants center around the improved psychological and sexual well-being of the patient after undergoing augmentation or reconstructive breast surgery. Enhanced self-image, self-esteem, and a high level of satisfaction are common feelings among patients.

It is recommended that all patients be made aware of the known risks, as well as the current concerns about potential risks, and that each individual patient, along with her surgeon, make a decision about the use of any type of implant. When applicable, it is hoped that the surgeon and patient will both participate in the collection of data to help determine the safety of these devices.

The Implant Operation

External scars that can result from augmentation are a concern of most patients. A variety of incisions can be used to accomplish placement of implants (Fig. 11-3). The most popular is the *submammary approach* in which a 4-cm curvilinear incision is made just above the inframammary crease. The scar is hidden by the inferior pole of the breast as it drapes. Some women prefer to have the scar hidden in the normal irregularities of the areola. A periareolar incision can be made through the inferior circumference of this pigmented tissue. An *axillary approach* can also be used. Previous scars also make convenient incision points for implant placement. Some experience is being reported with endoscopic placement of implants using incisions hidden in the umbilical region. To date there has not been widespread acceptance of this technique.

Fig. 11-3. Surgical incisions used in augmentation mammaplasty. Although the submammary approach is the most common, periareolar and axillary approaches are also used.

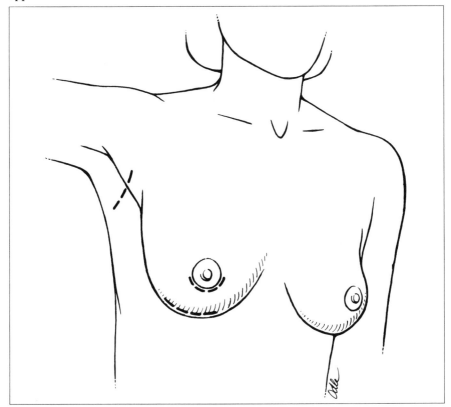

Implants can be placed either in a subglandular (also called subcutaneous or prepectoral) or submuscular (also called subpectoral) location (Fig. 11-4). For the subglandular implant, the interface between the breast parenchyma and the pectoralis fascia is dissected and the implant is placed in this pocket. For submuscular placement the pectoralis major muscle is dissected off the chest wall along with slips of the serratus and rectus muscles. The implant is then placed beneath this muscular cover.

The preferred location of the implant depends on the patient's history and body habitus (Table 11-2). Women with ptotic breasts or hypertrophic pectoral muscles are not good candidates for submuscular implant placement. Submuscular implants are not usually felt but can occasionally be seen in women with well-developed pectoralis muscles; contraction of these muscles may temporarily make the outline of the implant visible. In a woman with a minimal amount of native breast tissue, a subglandular implant may be more easily palpated, and creases or folds in the implant surface may be mistaken for masses on physical examination. Women who are at high risk for breast cancer (i.e., family history, precancerous biopsy) should have submuscular placement of implants; this facilitates the performance of screening mammography.

After implant placement, the size, shape, and symmetry are evaluated as the tissues are allowed to redrape over the implant intraoperatively. The patient is usually placed in a soft dressing and bra that is worn for several weeks to help mold the implant into its new breast pockets. Some patients are asked to perform exercises to "massage" the implants in the hope that this will help maintain the pocket diameter.

Almost all augmentations are performed on an outpatient basis. Local anesthesia with intravenous sedation is routine when the subglandular approach is chosen. When implants are placed submuscularly, general anesthesia is often preferred to facilitate muscle relaxation during surgery.

Complications

Immediate postoperative complications of implant placement include hematoma or seroma formation and peri-implant or incisional infection. Aspiration of fluid may be necessary to treat a hematoma or seroma, and a second surgical procedure is necessary occasionally to drain the fluid and replace the implant. An infection usually necessitates the administration of an antibiotic and the removal of the implant until the inflammatory process resolves.

Later complications of augmentation include capsular contracture, implant rupture with extravasation of silicone gel into soft tissues, contained rupture or deflation of the implant, focal herniations of the implant through the capsule, and altered breast sensation.

Formation of a fibrous capsule around the implant occurs in all

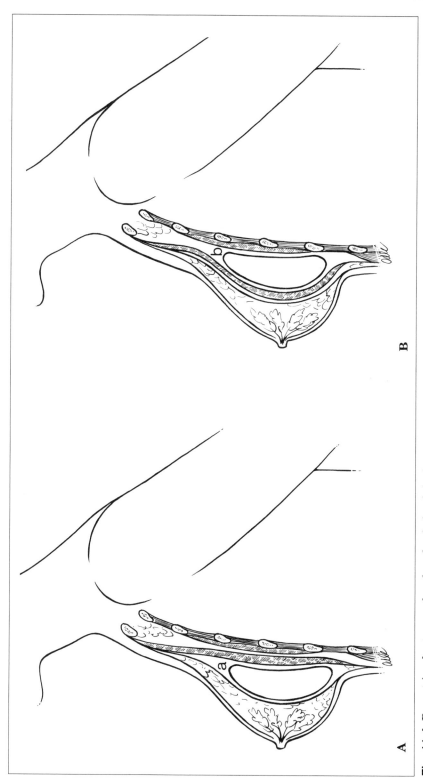

Fig. 11-4. Breast implants may be placed subglandularly (A) in the tissue plane anterior to the pectoralis muscle or submuscularly (B) beneath the pectoralis major muscle.

women as a normal physiologic response to the placement of a foreign body. In some women the capsule may become firm and palpable. The capsule may become visible as it causes tethering of the implant to the surrounding soft tissues. There may be distortion of the breast with movement of the breast tissue or underlying musculature (Fig. 11-5). Such changes are referred to as *capsular contracture*. Calcifications may also be deposited in the peri-implant capsule, leading to greater firmness of the capsule.

Capsular contractures are seen more frequently in patients with subglandular placement of implants. It is thought that submuscular placement results in fewer cases of capsular contracture due to the massaging action of the pectoral muscles as they contract and relax.

The traditional treatment for capsular contracture is a closed capsulotomy. For this procedure the patient is awake in clinic (occasionally lightly sedated). The surgeon forcefully compresses the fibrous capsule and implant by hand. This creates a "tear" in the capsule and allows the implant pocket to return to its original size and shape. When the fibrous capsule cannot be externally ruptured, it may be necessary to perform an open capsulotomy; the implant

Table 11-2. Preferred implant location by patient characteristics

Subglandular	Submuscular
Ptotic breasts	Minimal native breast tissue
Well-developed pectoral muscles	Postmastectomy (for reconstruction)
Moderate amount of native breast tissue	History of capsular contracture
	High risk for breast cancer

Fig. 11-5. Patient with a right breast capsular contracture 20 years after subglandular augmentation mammaplasty. Note the distorted skin and subcutaneous tissues produced by the fibrotic capsule surrounding the implant.

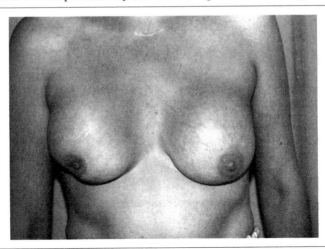

pocket is approached surgically and scoring/releasing incisions are made in the capsule under direct vision. In more severe cases of capsule formation the woman and her surgeon may elect to perform a capsulectomy to surgically remove the entire capsule around the implant (Fig. 11-6). The original implant can then be replaced or exchanged for a new implant.

Implant rupture may result from trauma, either blunt or penetrating. Such trauma may be iatrogenic because it occurs when closed capsulotomies are performed to relieve capsular contractures. If silicone gel implants have been used, implant rupture can result in extravasation of gel into the surrounding soft tissues and lymphatics. Alternatively, the gel may remain contained within the fibrous capsule that was formed around the intact implant. Although such a contained rupture usually leads to a change in the implanted breast's shape without a change in its volume, some contained ruptures of silicone gel implants are clinically inapparent. Rupture of a saline-containing implant leads to an acute decrease in breast volume as well as to a change in shape because the saline is readily absorbed by the surrounding tissue (Fig. 11-7). Removal of the implant is recommended after any type of rupture.

A tear in the surrounding fibrous capsule may also permit herniation of an intact implant through the capsule. On physical examination a mass may be felt on the implant surface where the herniation has occurred.

The life expectancy of implants is unknown but they cannot be

Fig. 11-6. On the right is an implant removed 25 years after subglandular placement. On the left is the surgical specimen of the fibrotic capsule that had formed around the implant. Note that the capsule is smaller than the implant. This is, in part, what causes the altered breast shape sometimes seen with severe capsular contractures.

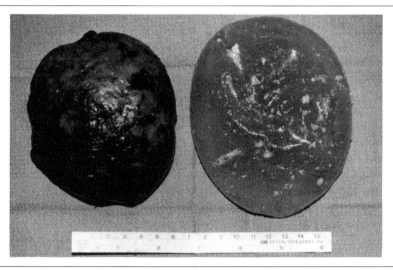

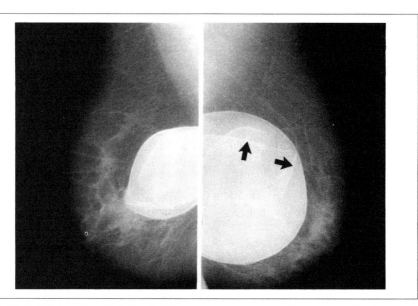

Fig. 11-7. Bilateral mediolateral oblique mammograms of a woman who has subglandular saline implants. Most of the saline in the right implant has leaked into the breast tissues where it has been absorbed, causing the right breast size to be reduced. Note normal folds *(arrows)* in the left implant.

considered lifetime devices. Prospective implant candidates should be made aware of this. The type of implant used and the lifestyle of the patient may influence implant longevity.

Lactation is not affected by augmentation mammaplasty because the milk ducts are not severed during the dissection. There have been reports, however, of traces of silicone and silicone antibodies in the breast milk of women with silicone implants. No adverse effects on the nursing infant have yet been reported. Breast size and shape will change after pregnancy despite the presence of an implant, and the mature breast shape seen postpartum may lead the patient to seek further breast surgery (i.e., mastopexy) to once again obtain a more youthful breast profile.

After augmentation surgery the plastic surgeon will usually follow the patient at regular intervals during the first year. Subsequent visits can be arranged if there are questions or concerns. Clinical diagnoses of complications are based primarily on the history elicited from the patient and on the physical examination. Patients should be advised to report any change in the size or shape of their breasts to their physician. Direct trauma to the breasts should also prompt a physical examination. Any suspicion of complications should prompt an investigative work-up.

Imaging of Implant Complications

A great deal of recent attention has been focused on the use of imaging techniques in assessing implant complications. Mammography, magnetic resonance imaging, and ultrasound are all useful. The optimal imaging algorithm has not yet been determined but when an implant complication is suspected clinically, and imaging is desired, an experienced facility should be sought. The radiologist should be given as much clinical information as possible so that he or she can tailor the work-up to be as safe, efficient, and inexpensive as possible.

MAMMOGRAPHY. Experience has shown that mammography alone can detect many implant complications. Fibrous encapsulation can be visualized, particularly in women with subglandular positioning of their implants. Herniation of an intact implant through a tear in the fibrous capsule can also be seen mammographically, although special views may be required. Implant rupture with extracapsular extravasation of silicone can also be detected mammographically (Fig. 11-8). Recent reports have shown that clinically unsuspected rupture of silicone implants is visualized in 5% of women with implants who present for screening mammography. The proportion of extracapsular ruptures not seen mammographically is unknown. It is possible that when only a small amount of silicone has extravasated it may be obscured on the mammogram by the implant's overlying density.

MAGNETIC RESONANCE IMAGING. Magnetic resonance imaging is the most sensitive and specific modality for detection of silicone implant rupture. Extravasated silicone can be visualized in the breast parenchyma, in the axilla, and in the muscles. Intracapsular ruptures can also be detected, and in such ruptures the silicone is contained within the fibrous capsule that was formed around the implant (Fig. 11-9). Intracapsular implant ruptures are difficult to detect using mammography. There are unanswered questions about the clinical significance of these contained ruptures, but current policy is to recommend removal. Their significance may lie in the possibility of conversion to an extracapsular rupture by manual closed capsulotomy or by compression during mammography. Free silicone gel also may be able to permeate the capsule.

ULTRASOUND. Ultrasound is a less expensive screening tool for the detection of intracapsular or extracapsular implant rupture. Extravasated silicone is identifiable by ultrasound provided that it is located in the area examined. Intracapsular implant ruptures are also reported to have a characteristic ultrasound appearance, but the sensitivity and specificity of this technique in the detection of implant ruptures are lower than magnetic resonance imaging. Additional comparative studies of these imaging modalities are needed so that their respective roles in the detection of implant complications can be clarified.

Other areas of controversy in the management of the patient with breast implants include the advisability of radiologic screening for implant complications. Routine screening in women who are asymptomatic or in women who are not old enough to warrant mammo-

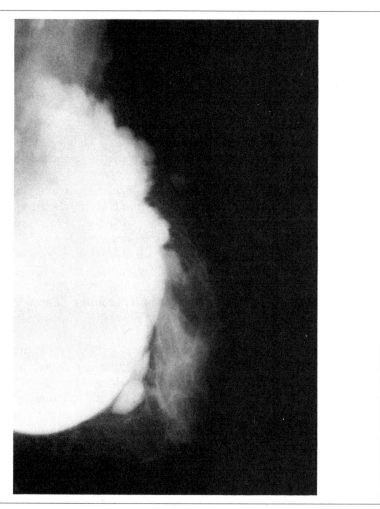

Fig. 11-8. A left subglandular silicone implant that has ruptured. The silicone has extravasated into the soft tissue of the breast and axilla.

graphic screening for breast cancer is not currently advised, but may be requested by women who are aware of the risk of rupture.

Removal of Implants (Explantation)

In the wake of the intense media coverage of the controversy surrounding the silicone gel implant, many women have consulted with their physicians regarding the possibility of removing their implants or exchanging them for a "safer" implant. For some women this desire to be rid of the silicone gel has resulted in a panic state for which nothing short of explantation will suffice. For others simply exchanging the silicone gel implant for a saline one provides relief from their anxiety.

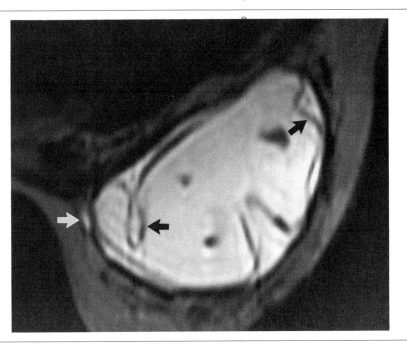

Fig. 11-9. Spin Echo (SE) T2 weighted, water-suppressed magnetic resonance image of the right breast showing an intracapsular implant rupture. The wavy black lines *(black arrows)* represent the collapsed shell of the implant floating within the extravasated silicone that is now contained within the fibrous capsule. Medially, there is also a small area of extracapsular silicone *(white arrow)*.

Multiple problems arise when requests for explantation or exchange are made. Because the breast skin has been stretched to accommodate its new volume, the simple removal of the implant will potentially leave a flaccid skin envelope with ptosis and a flattened profile. For the many women who initially sought augmentation to enhance their breasts, this may result in an unacceptable breast shape. The shape can be retained if they desire to have another implant placed, but for those who desire to be silicone-free the only choice is breast reconstruction. Surgical procedures to remove the implants expose the patient to further risks of anesthesia, blood loss, and loss of breast tissue. To remove the implants and their capsule, a small rim of breast tissue adherent to the capsule is removed, leading to a small loss in breast volume. If the capsules are particularly firm and difficult to remove, a risk of blood loss, perhaps necessitating blood replacement, exists. Postoperative complications are similar to those for other surgical procedures with the added disadvantage of a possible poor aesthetic result.

Concurrent procedures to reshape the breast can be performed; a mastopexy reshapes the breast envelope leaving the remaining parenchyma intact, or muscle flaps can be used to fill in the additional volume desired for breast contour.

Monetary considerations are an issue for many women who may have a different financial picture at the time they desire explantation than when they first paid for the augmentation procedure. General anesthesia is often necessary for successful explantation and this costs significantly more than the usual global fee for implantation. Some manufacturers have offered to help defray these costs, but not all women qualify for these benefits. This has led many women to seek assistance from the legal community in order to recoup some of their monetary outlay.

Current recommendations for explantation are to remove those implants that are either ruptured, have a deformed, painful capsule, or cause significant emotional distress for the patient. Routine removal or exchange of implants is not justified by scientific evidence.

Patients who are experiencing symptoms that they believe to be related to their implants may continue to experience these same symptoms (i.e., fatigue, malaise, weight loss, memory loss, hair loss, skin dryness, pain) after the implants have been removed. There is a small population of women, however, who have experienced attenuation of their symptomatology with explantation. Whether this is from any actual benefit derived from the silicone removal or from their reduced anxiety level is uncertain.

Breast Cancer Screening in the Augmented Breast

Women who have undergone breast augmentation are not at increased risk for developing breast cancer nor are they immune to it. Adherence to the American Cancer Society breast cancer screening guidelines (see Chap. 4) is suggested for women with breast implants. It is, of course, undeniable that both clinical and mammographic screening are more difficult in these women.

Performance of mammography after augmentation requires special expertise. Women should be referred to radiology facilities that are familiar with examination of women with implants. It is preferable that a radiologist be on site both to review films for technical quality and also to answer any questions that the patient may have. Examination of the augmented breast is more time consuming, therefore the radiology office should be informed of the presence of implants when the mammogram is scheduled.

A screening mammogram of the augmented breast usually begins with the two standard mammographic views using moderate compression. A 90-degree lateral film may also be taken in women with subglandular implants. These views are followed by implant displacement or Eklund views (i.e., craniocaudal and mediolateral oblique) during which the implant is manually pushed posteriorly

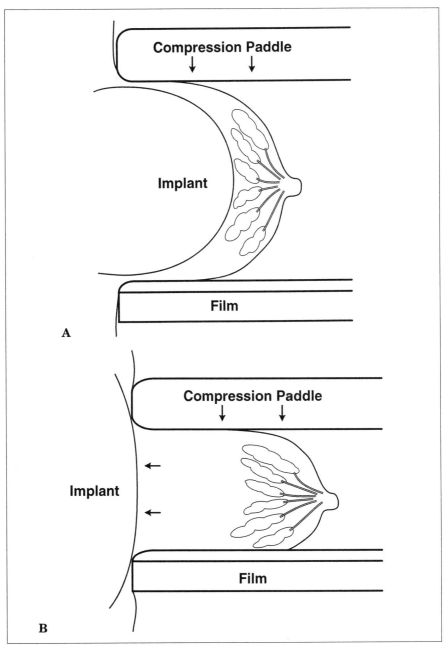

Fig. 11-10. Schematic drawing showing how mammography is performed in the augmented breast. Standard views (A) are taken first and the implant is compressed with moderate force. Implant displacement views (B) are performed while the implant is pushed posteriorly against the chest wall and the compression plate is firmly applied to the native tissue anteriorly.

against the chest wall while the compression plate is firmly applied to the native tissue anterior to the implant (Figs. 11-10 and 11-11).

The vulnerability of implants to rupture during mammographic compression is unknown. No documented cases of such ruptures have been reported. In vitro studies have shown that compressive force far greater than that used in clinical mammography is required to rupture new, unused implants. However, as implants age in vivo they may become more fragile.

Even when implant displacement views are added, an average of about 25% of the breast is not imaged on routine screening in women with implants because all implant devices are radiopaque. Implant location determines to a great degree how much breast tissue is seen. Submuscular implants provide greater visualization of native tissue than do subglandular implants. Only about 15% of breast tissue is not seen with submuscular placement, whereas with subglandular placement, tissue visualization is reduced by about 35%. Capsular contracture can severely limit mammographic visualization of native tissue both because it is difficult to obtain adequate compression for standard views and because the implants cannot be displaced posteriorly for adequate viewing of the anterior native tissue (Fig. 11-12). Visualization of breast tissue on mammograms in women who have severe capsular contractures may be reduced by as much as 50%.

Although there are no large-scale studies demonstrating decreased mammographic sensitivity after augmentation, it is safe to assume that there is some reduction in our ability to discover breast cancer in its earliest stage in women who have breast implants, particularly if they are subglandular in location. Women should be counseled as such before undergoing augmentation.

Despite these limitations, screening mammography can successfully diagnose many cases of occult breast cancer in the augmented breast. Women with implants should receive the same attention to breast cancer screening as other women so that when malignancy is diagnosed it is less likely to be at an advanced stage.

Other Contour-Altering Procedures

Mastopexy and reduction mammaplasty are other breast contour-altering procedures routinely performed by plastic surgeons.

Mastopexy

For a mastopexy, the skin of the breast is reduced by separating it from the underlying parenchyma. The redundant skin is excised, and a smaller breast skin envelope is created. This corrects problems such as postlactational and involutional macromastia and ptosis. The nipple is elevated back to its youthful position opposite the infra-

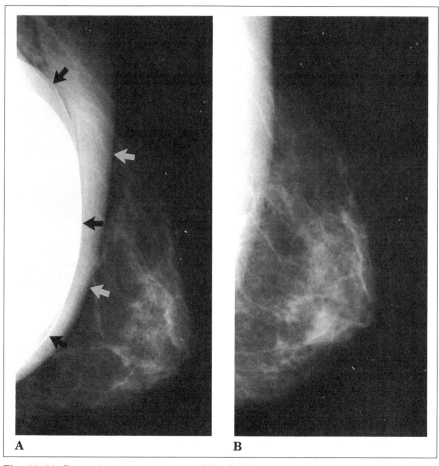

A   B

Fig. 11-11. Screening mammogram of the left breast in a woman with submuscular double-lumen implants. On the standard mediolateral oblique view (A) the implant *(black arrows)* is seen beneath the pectoralis major muscle *(white arrows)*. On the mediolateral oblique displacement view (B), the compression paddle is brought down so that the implant is displaced posteriorly (out of view). Note the greater detail (due to better compression) seen in the native tissues on the displacement view.

mammary fold. No change in the actual breast volume or function is attained with this technique.

Reduction Mammaplasty

A reduction mammaplasty involves excision of both excess breast parenchyma and skin as well as a repositioning of the nipple-areolar complex. The volume of breast tissue removed ranges from a few hundred grams to more than 2000 grams. A breast size that is proportional to the patient's body habitus is the goal of reduction mammaplasty. The patient is frequently reduced to a B or C cup. Can-

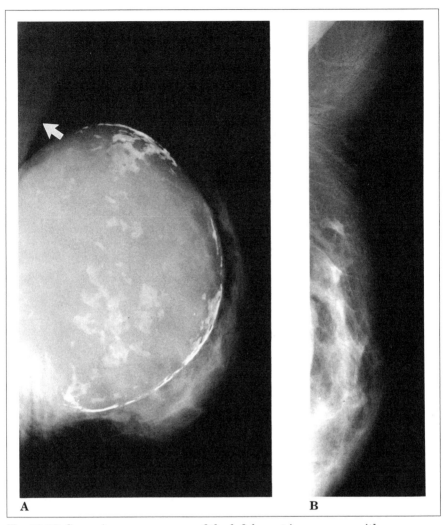

Fig. 11-12. Screening mammogram of the left breast in a woman with subglandular implants. There is extensive calcification in the fibrous capsule surrounding the implant on the standard view (A). The pectoralis major muscle *(white arrow)* passes posterior to the implant. On the displacement view (B) a limited amount of native tissue is visualized anterior to the implant. Subglandular implants do not displace as far posteriorly as submuscular implants.

didates for this procedure often have enormous breasts resulting from macromastia, postpartum changes, or weight gain. The extreme weight of the breasts elicits problems of neck pain, shoulder grooving, and occasionally paresthesias in the brachial plexus. No relation to pulmonary dysfunction has been demonstrated. Unfortunately, while the surgeon is often able to sympathize with such patients, many insurance carriers do not. Unless it can be documented by neurologic testing that nerve impairment exists, this operative procedure is rarely covered by a third-party payer.

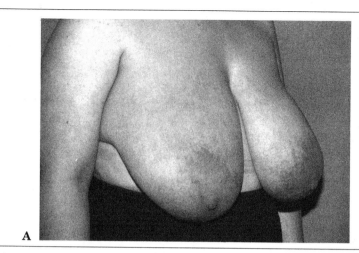

Fig. 11-13. A. Preoperative patient with macromastia seen in consultation for reduction mammaplasty.

Breast reduction is a relatively complex operation necessitating general anesthesia and autologous blood donation. The tissue that is excised is routinely sent for pathologic examination, and up to 4% of specimens may contain occult premalignant or malignant changes. All patients over age 30 should have preoperative mammographic screening. Complications from reduction surgery are the same as with other surgical procedures (e.g., hematoma, infection). There also may be loss of sensation to the breast, nipple, and/or areola; this may include loss of erectile function. The patient's ability to lactate may also be lost; however, the risk of this loss can be minimized by using certain surgical approaches (e.g., inferior pedicle technique). Thus, if a patient is particularly concerned about loss of lactation it should be discussed preoperatively with the plastic surgeon. The skin flaps are also at risk for partial loss, and the visible scars tend to widen with time. Nevertheless, reduction mammaplasty patients tend to be exceptionally happy with their altered breast contour (Fig. 11-13).

Women who have undergone reduction mammaplasty should follow the American Cancer Society guidelines for breast cancer screening. When a postreduction patient presents for mammography it is important that the radiologist be aware of the patient's surgical history. A variety of postreduction mammographic changes are noted. These include architectural distortion, parenchymal displacement, skin thickening, dystrophic calcifications, and fat necrosis. Sequential mammograms help document the stability of these postsurgical changes to avoid unnecessary biopsies. The location of mammographic findings seen on prereduction films may change. Patients should be reminded to bring previous studies from other institutions

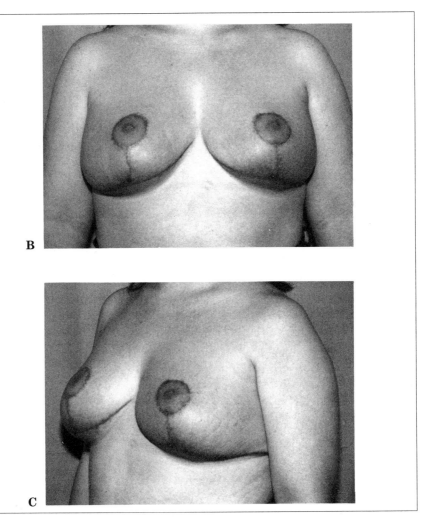

Fig. 11-13. (continued) B, C. The same patient in the early postoperative period after reduction mammaplasty. Note the position of the scars from the incisions used for this technique.

to the current radiology facility to avoid delay in interpretation of their mammograms.

Suggested Reading

Biggs TM, and Humphreys DH. Augmentation mammaplasty. In Smith JW, Aston SJ (eds). *Plastic Surgery* (4th ed). Boston: Little, Brown, 1991. Pp 1145–1156.

Destouet JM, et al. Screening mammography in 350 women with breast implants: Prevalence and findings of implant complications. *AJR* 159:973, 1992.

Everson LI, et al. Diagnosis of breast implant rupture: Imaging findings and relative efficacies of imaging techniques. *AJR* 163:57, 1994.

Gabriel SE, et al. Risk of connective tissue diseases and other disorders after breast implantation. *N Engl J Med* 330:1697, 1994.

Gorczyca DP, et al. Silicone breast implants in vivo: MR imaging. *Radiology* 185:407, 1992.

Handel N, Silverstein MJ, and Gamagami P. Factors affecting mammographic visualization of the breast after augmentation mammaplasty. *JAMA* 268:1913, 1992.

Kessler DA. Special Report. The basis of the FDA's decision on breast implants. *N Engl J Med* 326:1713, 1992.

Kossovsky N, Heggers JP, and Robson MC. The bioreactivity of silicone. In DF Williams (ed). *CRC Critical Reviews in Biocompatibility,* Volume 3. Boca Raton, FL: CRC Press, 1987. Pp 53–85.

Little JW, Spear SL, and Romm S. Reduction mammaplasty and mastopexy. In JW Smith, SJ Aston (eds). *Plastic Surgery* (4th ed). Boston: Little, Brown, 1991. Pp 1157–1202.

Silverstein MJ, et al. Breast cancer diagnosis and prognosis in women augmented with silicone gel-filled implants. *Cancer* 66:97, 1990.

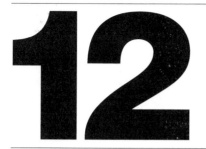

The High-Risk Patient

Lois F. O'Grady
and Mary B. Rippon

The factors that have been identified as increasing a woman's risk of breast cancer have been discussed in Chaps. 2, 3, and 4.

Risk is reported in several ways, and, thus, a few words of explanation are in order. The *absolute risk* is based on population and can be expressed as cases per 100,000 or, more commonly, by the cumulative or lifetime risk. *Cumulative risk* assumes that all patients have the same risk and that the population will all live to be a certain age. For breast cancer, this means that 1 in 10 women will develop cancer if the population lives to be 80 years of age. If one assumes that the population will live longer, for example, to age 85 or 100, the risk goes up to 1 in 9 or 1 in 8, respectively, because the entire population is living longer and has more time to develop a cancer. Such figures are an overestimate for women with no risk factors and an underestimate for women with risk factors.

A more meaningful estimate of risk is the relative risk (RR), that is, What is the patient's risk compared to a woman who has absolutely no risk factors? A woman who has absolutely no risk factors other than her gender has a 3.3% chance of developing breast cancer some time in her life. For example, a study that reports that drinking alcohol carries an RR of 1.2, means that the risk is 1.2 times the 3.3%, or 3.96%.

High-Risk Factors

The three factors (other than increasing age) that significantly increase the risk of breast cancer are prior breast cancer, strong family history, and atypical hyperplasia on biopsy (Table 12-1).

Table 12-1. Major risk factors for breast cancer

Risk factor	Chance of developing breast cancer (%)
Prior breast cancer	20
Strong family history	6–18
Atypical hyperplasia	16–33

Previous History of Breast Cancer

Once a woman has had breast cancer, she has a 20% chance of developing cancer in the other breast. From the time of diagnosis, this risk increases at 0.8% per year until the 20% risk is reached.

Strong Family History

A strong family history can be defined as two or more first-degree (i.e., mother, sister) relatives with breast cancer. A woman whose mother had breast cancer has an RR of 1.8, a woman whose sister had breast cancer carries an RR of 2.5, and if both mother and sister had breast cancer the RR is 5.6. The actual risk can be calculated by multiplying the baseline risk, 3.3%, by the RR factor. The RR figures above translate into 6%, 8%, and 18% for actual risk. If the cancers in the family occur prior to the menopause, or if they tend to occur bilaterally, the risk increases. In all probability, the risk never exceeds 35%.

Molecular biologists are within months of identifying the precise location of one of the genes that control some familial breast cancers. It lies on chromosome 17, and it appears that the gene can be passed through paternal lineage. This exciting development is expected to lead to a genetic probe that can screen known breast cancer families to determine which women in the family carry the excess risk. It is important to keep this in perspective, however, because only 10% of breast cancers are of the hereditary type and not all will manifest the gene.

Atypical Hyperplasia

A number of studies have shown that women who harbor atypical hyperplastic changes in the breast have an increased risk of breast cancer. With no family history, the RR is about 5, or 16% ($5 \times 3.3\% = 16\%$). In the face of a positive family history of cancer, the RR is 11 or 33% ($11 \times 3.3\% = 33\%$). Note that this figure is close to the theoretical 35% mentioned above.

Lobular carcinoma in situ is a special type of atypical hyperplastic disease (see Chap. 13) and is associated with an increased risk of cancer *in either breast,* and of ductal or lobular character. The risk is strikingly similar to that of a patient with a previous history of cancer—1% per year to a maximum of about 25%.

These factors, then, define a population of patients who, because of their relatively high risk, deserve special consideration in terms of counseling, monitoring, and prevention. Although these patients have a higher risk of cancer, it must be stressed that the cancers that develop in these patients are in no way unusual. They are not easier or harder to detect, nor are they more aggressive or harder to treat.

Monitoring for Cancer Detection

The basic tools for detection of breast cancer remain self-examination by the patient, examination by the practitioner, and mammography. Table 12-2 shows the frequency with which the examinations should be performed in these high-risk groups.

Mammography should be able to detect 85% to 90% of cancers when they are 1 cm or less in size, providing that the screening is done annually. However, the density of the breast, the radiographic character of the tumor, and technical factors limit the sensitivity of this technique (see Chap. 4).

In theory, careful physical examination of a normal breast by a professional can detect a tumor at about 1 cm, but tumors are usually in the 2-cm range when detected. The size of the breast, its density, and its nodularity limit the sensitivity of physical examination.

Examination by the patient is not usually as accurate but has the advantage of detecting tumors that appear between physician examinations. Women should be encouraged to consult their physicians for assessment of any change in their breasts regardless of how recently they had a negative mammogram or examination.

Prevention Strategies

Cancer prevention strategies are grouped into three general categories:

1. Elimination of risk factors
2. Behavior modification
3. Preventive agent (tamoxifen)

Elimination of Risk Factors

The cause of any cancer is multifactorial, and breast cancer is no exception. Unlike lung cancer and skin cancer in which the major risk factors (smoking and sun exposure) can be eliminated, the major risk factors for breast cancer—genetic makeup, age, and a previous history of cancer—cannot be altered. Although we know many minor factors that are associated with the risk of breast cancer, there is

Table 12-2. Monitoring frequency for high-risk patients

Procedure	Frequency
Breast self-examination	Monthly
Physician breast examination	Every 4 months
Mammography	Yearly

scant evidence available to show whether altering these factors can alter the risk.

Behavior Modification

Diet
The lay and semiscientific press hold that a low-fat diet, maintenance of body weight near ideal, and avoidance of alcohol can reduce risk. These may be admirable goals, and it makes intuitive sense that they would help, but no strong evidence exists to support these claims. Some of the factors that incite breast cancer may occur 10 to 20 years prior to diagnosis. If dietary changes are ever to be effective as a preventative measure, they may well have to be initiated in childhood and then maintained for life.

A 13-year study funded by the National Institutes of Health and the Women's Health Initiative began in 1993. It will focus on whether a low-fat diet can reduce the incidence of breast cancer.

Hormonal Changes
Hormonal changes that occur through childbearing and the use of hormonal therapy influence the incidence of breast cancer (see Chaps. 3 and 10). A woman's choice of if and when she bears a child and her choice of whether to use postmenopausal hormone therapy can influence her risk of breast cancer. Because a woman can decide whether or when to have a child and whether to use hormone therapy, these choices are mentioned here under behavior modification.

Late age at first birth or nulliparity are known risk factors for breast cancer. It is known also that early surgical menopause protects against breast cancer. There is some suggestion that part of the increased incidence of breast cancer in affluent countries is related to a prolonged menstrual life. Better nutrition (perhaps too good) leads to earlier menarche. More women in so-called advanced countries are delaying childbearing until later years; thus, there is a population of women whose breasts undergo 20 or more years of cyclic stimulation before coming to full maturation, that is, lactation.

Some argue that women known to be at higher risk for breast cancer should bear a child in their teens to alter this cycle. Despite any sense that this might make, it must be stressed that the theory is just that, a theory, and that there is no proof that early childbearing will change appreciably the risk for any one woman.

No one has addressed the question of deliberate oophorectomy to reduce risk.

The issue of estrogen use and breast cancer is discussed in Chap. 10. It is probably prudent for women at high risk of developing breast cancer to avoid estrogen replacement therapy. After weighing the risks and benefits, however, some women do elect to take postmenopausal estrogens for a few years.

The possible risk of oral contraceptive use has received much attention through the years. Some studies have shown an increased risk, many have shown no increased risk, and some have shown a protective effect. Almost all of the studies have been flawed in some way. If oral contraceptives are a risk at all, it is a minimal risk. Not enough evidence exists to advise patients to avoid their use.

Preventive Agent

Tamoxifen

In an ideal world, it would be best to prevent breast cancer rather than try to detect it once it has formed. In Chaps. 8 and 15, the use of an antiestrogen, tamoxifen, in treating fibrocystic disease and in preventing relapses of breast cancer is discussed. In the laboratory, this drug has been shown to inhibit the growth and development of breast cancer cells. In the large tamoxifen studies done in the United States and in Great Britain, the incidence of second cancers was lower among the treated women. In fact, the incidence of second cancers was decreased by almost 40%.

Because of these findings, and because of the relative safety of the drug, there are major studies under way in the United States and Europe using tamoxifen as a chemopreventive agent. The studies use rigid criteria to define high risk and randomize patients to receive tamoxifen or a placebo for 5 years.

We know that there is a long period in the life of a breast cancer, perhaps as long as 10 to 12 years, before it can be detected. It is not known definitively whether the tamoxifen actually prevents the development of the second cancers, or whether it just slows down the rate of growth such that these second cancers will appear later. The preventive effect of the drug was maintained after the drug was stopped, however, leading to the assumption that it was preventing cancer rather than just slowing the growth.

It will be many years before the results of the studies are known. At the present time, physicians dealing with these high-risk patients are caught between their "physician-scientist" side that dictates that no patient should be given the drug until the results of the studies are available, and their "compassionate physician" side that does not like to deny a potentially beneficial treatment to a patient.

The drug is not without some risk and should not be given routinely without careful assessment.

There are no other chemopreventive agents available at this time.

Mastectomy

In theory, one sure way to prevent breast cancer would be to remove the breasts. Prophylactic total mastectomy, with or without reconstruction, and subcutaneous mastectomy have been used to treat both women with severe mastalgia and women at high risk for breast cancer. Each procedure has its proponents and its drawbacks which need to be taken into consideration before addressing the decision of whether to have surgery.

The Procedure

Proponents of prophylactic total mastectomy or subcutaneous mastectomy suggest that these procedures eliminate the risk of cancer. At best they reduce the risk; *neither* procedure removes *all* of the breast tissue. Total mastectomy leaves glandular tissue in the inframammary areas and in the superficial layers of the pectoralis fascia muscle. Subcutaneous mastectomy, in addition, leaves glandular tissue in the skin and nipple-areolar complex.

Plastic surgeons often prefer the subcutaneous procedure because of better cosmesis. Surgical oncologists decry the procedure as inadequate for cancer control.

Both procedures are permanent and deforming. Patients need to be aware that, as with any reconstruction using implants, there is a risk of cosmetically unacceptable encapsulation with fibrous tissue and subsequent distortion. An occasional patient does not tolerate the implants and removal becomes necessary. In addition, subcutaneous mastectomy frequently alters the sensation to the nipple-areolar complex.

The Decision

The decision of whether to have prophylactic mastectomy is not an easy one and should never be made in haste. At all times, it is important to remember that cancers grow slowly and that surgery leads to a permanent loss.

Most often, patients begin to consider prophylactic mastectomy when a second or third near (i.e., first-degree) relative is diagnosed with cancer or dies from it. Because both the patient and the family can be distraught, this is not the best time to make irrevocable decisions. It is the time for information gathering, for careful discussion of the options, and for a 6-month period of reflection.

The factors that must be addressed include (1) the exact risk of cancer in the family, (2) the ease with which the patient's breasts can be palpated, (3) the ease with which mammograms can be read, and, equally important, (4) the psychological state of the patient (Table 12-3).

Table 12-3. Factors to consider before prophylactic mastectomy

Cancer risk
Physical examination
Mammographic pattern
Psychological state

A well-informed oncologist should be able to provide a patient with a reasonable assessment of risk. In some cities special genetic counseling centers are available.

The more dense and nodular the breast, the more difficult it will be to detect a developing cancer by physical examination. If the breast is equally dense radiographically, the sensitivity of mammography will be decreased. The ease or difficulty of cancer detection will be an important component of the decision tree.

A careful assessment of the psychological status of the patient is critical and must be made at a time distant from acute breast cancer crises in the family. It is important to assess the degree of cancer fear, whether these fears and concerns are rational, and whether that fear is interfering significantly with the patient's life.

A patient whose breasts are easy to examine, physically and radiographically, and who is not overwhelmed by cancer risk, is a candidate for careful monitoring and not for surgery.

A patient whose breasts are difficult to examine, especially radiographically, and whose life is impacted significantly by her worry and concern, may be a candidate for prophylactic mastectomy. A 6-month period of reflection and consultation is recommended most strongly before final decisions are made.

Suggested Reading

Risk

Henderson IC. Risk factors for breast cancer. *Cancer* (suppl) 71: 2127–2140, 1993.

Kelly PT. *Understanding Breast Cancer Risk.* Philadelphia: Temple University Press, 1991.

Love SM. Use of risk factors in counseling patients. *Hematol Oncol Clin North Am* 3:599–610, 1989.

Chemoprevention

Atiba JO, and Meyskens FL. Chemoprevention of breast cancer. *Semin Oncol* 19:220–229, 1992.

Mastectomy

Goodnight JE, Quagliana JM, and Morton DL. Failure of subcutaneous mastectomy to prevent the development of breast cancer. *J Surg Oncol* 26:198–201, 1984.

Pennisi VR, and Capozzi A. Subcutaneous mastectomy data: A final statistical analysis of 1500 patients. *Aesthetic Plastic Surg* 13:15–21, 1989.

Temple WJ, et al. Technical considerations for prophylactic mastectomy in patients at high risk for breast cancer. *Am J Surg* 161:413–415, 1991.

Wapnir IL, Rabinowitz B, and Greco RS. A reappraisal of prophylactic mastectomy. *Surg Gynecol Obstet* 171:171–184, 1990.

Treatment
and Follow-Up

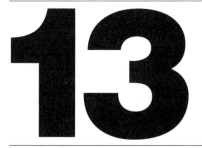

13

Atypical Hyperplasia and Carcinoma in Situ

Lois F. O'Grady,
Lydia Pleotis Howell,
and Mary B. Rippon

Atypical hyperplasia and carcinoma in situ represent the early phases of a continuum of morphologic change in the terminal duct lobular units (TDLUs) that may lead to invasive cancer. The TDLU is the structure that encompasses the very end of the branching duct system and the small lobule of glandular tissue it drains, and which is responsive to hormonal and carcinogenic influences (see Chaps. 1 and 2). The malignant process may begin as simple hyperplasia, proceed to atypical hyperplastic changes, and then to carcinoma in situ of either the ductal or lobular type (Fig. 13-1). Regardless of where it begins in the TDLU (Fig. 13-2), the malignancy can spread up and down the ductal-lobular tree, sometimes traveling great distances before becoming an infiltrating cancer. The process evolves over a considerable time span of 10, 15, or even 20 years. When a patient has a breast biopsy, the picture reported by the pathologist, and the patient's subsequent risk, depend entirely on the lesion's location in that continuum.

Twenty years ago these noninvasive lesions were rare (less than 5% of cancers), but with increasingly sophisticated medicine and the increased use of mammography and biopsy, as well as other unknown factors, we are seeing many more of these lesions. Recent reviews show carcinomas in situ to comprise up to 25% of newly diagnosed cancers (25% of those detected mammographically and 5% of those detected clinically). Considerable difference exists in the significance of the type of carcinoma in situ, in the way that they are found, and in the way that they are treated.

The understanding of hyperplasia, atypical hyperplasia, and carcinoma in situ, and consensus on the management of the latter two lesions are still evolving.

Hyperplasia

If hyperplastic changes alone are seen on biopsy, there is no way to know whether these changes are premalignant or not. The majority, by far, are not. This is reflected in the low risk of breast cancer that exists in those patients who have only hyperplastic changes seen on biopsy. It is mentioned here to emphasize that it is not the same

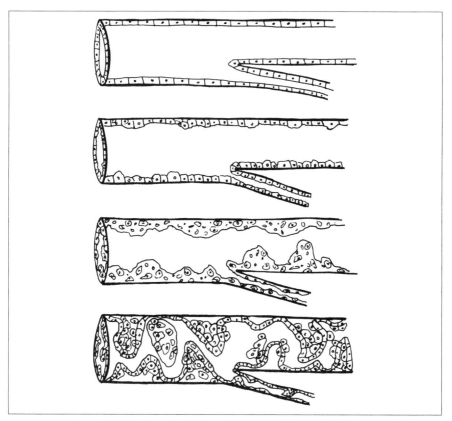

Fig. 13-1. Artist's representation of the breast duct lining showing *(top to bottom)* normal morphology, mild hyperplastic changes, atypical hyperplasia, and carcinoma in situ.

lesion as that addressed in the section on atypical hyperplasia that follows.

Atypical Hyperplasia

If the pathologist reports atypical hyperplastic changes, this should wave a red flag at the clinician because this breast is harboring changes that place it at high risk for cancer. The cancer can develop anywhere and in either breast. Is invasive cancer inevitable? No. Patients with atyical hyperplasia—about 4% of patients with fibrocystic changes—have a risk of breast cancer that is 4 to 5 times that of the general population. It is evident, therefore, that some of these lesions never progress or progress so slowly that the patient dies of other causes before the malignancy manifests itself. What stops this progression to malignancy? We don't really know. Some lesions recede with the menopause, and we think some recede with anties-

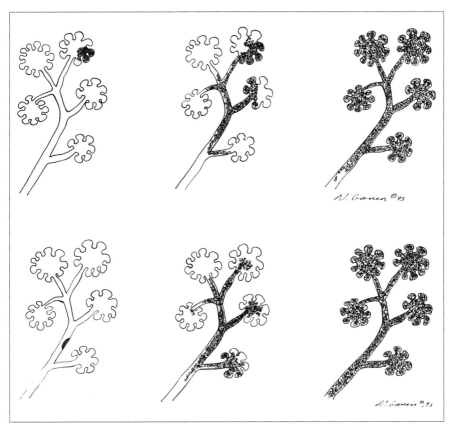

Fig. 13-2. Artist's representation of the spread of carcinoma in situ up and down the ductal-lobular system.

trogen therapy (see Chap. 12 on the high-risk patient), but we really do not know what controls the evolution toward malignancy.

Clinically, the patient with atypical hyperplasia is a high-risk patient and needs to be watched closely. She will require a careful, thorough examination by a health professional every 6 months; careful teaching of breast self-examination by that same health professional with frequent reinforcement and review of techniques; and yearly mammography.

If this patient has a family history of breast cancer, her risk doubles again—to 11 times that of the general population. She may be considered for a prevention protocol (see Chap. 12) or other types of prophylaxis such as mastectomy.

Carcinoma in Situ

If the pathologist reports the finding of carcinoma in situ, we know that the process is far along and, sooner or later, 30% of these patients (and probably more) will develop infiltrating cancers, which may not appear for 10 years.

There are two types of in situ cancer: lobular and ductal. Their clinical significance and treatment differ markedly.

Lobular Carcinoma in Situ

Lobular carcinoma in situ is usually an incidental finding on a breast biopsy done to investigate something else. It rarely forms a mass large enough to be palpable, and if it is palpable, the mass has a consistency like that of a normal breast. *Lobular carcinoma in situ does not show up on mammogram*—a most important clinical point. Interestingly, the incidence decreases considerably in postmenopausal women.

Most of these masses do not progress to infiltrating cancer. However, women who harbor lobular carcinoma in situ are at very high risk of developing an infiltrating cancer of either the lobular or ductal type in either breast any time over the next 10 to 15 years. These women must be placed in the "high risk, watch closely" group and may be considered for prophylactic intervention trials.

Therapeutically, the lesion may be excised with adequate margins. There is absolutely no indication for mastectomy and no need to search for metastatic disease. Large lesions should be reviewed carefully by the pathologist for the presence of elements of ductal carcinoma in situ because its presence changes the treatment recommendations.

Both breasts must be observed closely in a patient with a history of lobular carcinoma in situ. Physician examination should be performed every 4 months, and yearly mammography is indicated. Any changes in the breast or in the mammogram must be investigated promptly.

Ductal Carcinoma in Situ

Ductal carcinoma in situ (DCIS) is also referred to as an intraductal carcinoma and sometimes as a noninvasive cancer. It is a precursor to, but distinct from, infiltrating ductal carcinoma. It is very different from its lobular cousin and carries a more immediate risk to the patient.

Characteristics of DCIS
Some of these lesions develop calcifications when they are very small and are readily detected on mammography, whereas others present with large palpable lesions which are not well seen mammographically. We now know that there are two types: comedo type and noncomedo (sometimes called micropapillary or cribriform) type (Table 13-1).

Table 13-1. A comparison of ductal carcinomas in situ

	Comedo	Noncomedo
%	60	40
Architecture	Solid	Micropapillary/cribriform
Necrosis	Frequent	Rare
Calcification	95%	50%
Type calcification	Casting	Fine granular
Pathologic size vs. mammographic size	Slightly larger	Much larger
Nuclear grade	High	Low
Her-2-Neu oncogene	Present	Absent

The most important features of the *comedo type* are (1) it tends to become necrotic and therefore calcifies early; the calcifications are "casting" in type, mimicking a cast of the duct tree; (2) *the actual size of the lesion is very close to what is seen on the mammogram—a critical point for the surgeon;* and (3) it tends to have an aggressive clinical course.

In contrast, the *noncomedo* (cribriform or micropapillary) form (1) calcifies less often and when it does the calcifications are finely speckled; (2) is frequently not seen on mammography and when seen *the actual size does not necessarily correspond to the mammographic size* and may be much more extensive (again, critical information for planning biopsies); and (3) tends to be less aggressive clinically.

Therapeutic Principles

Twenty years ago, there was no discussion about the treatment of carcinoma in situ—patients had mastectomies. This treatment was 100% effective. There was rarely a recurrence, and no one died of the disease.

Today, however, the treatment seems excessively mutilating given that we now know that infiltrating cancer can be treated without removing the breast. The National Surgical Adjuvant Breast Project (NSABP) has done a study, the results of which showed that patients with infiltrating cancers have the same survival rates whether they are treated with total mastectomy, lumpectomy and radiation, or with lumpectomy alone. Although the latter group has a local recurrence rate of 35%, if the patient is watched closely for recurrence and treated appropriately, the survival rates are good.

Intuitively, then, one would presume that intraductal cancer, a less malignant process, could be treated conservatively also, and yet maintain the near 100% survivals, free of disease. In evaluating such conservative treatment regimens we have learned much about the biologic nature of the lesion, and reviewing these studies is instructive.

Excision Alone or with Radiotherapy?

When large trials of treatment for infiltrating cancers were reviewed, subsets of patients were identified with intraductal but not infiltrating cancers. From the reviews it appeared that these women did well with conservative therapy and had a high chance of disease-free survival.

Further studies have shown that excision alone is probably not adequate because there was a 20% to 25% local recurrence rate. While all these recurrences were local, half were of intraductal cancer and half were of infiltrating cancers with more ominous impact. In fact, a few patients who recurred with infiltrating cancers died of metastatic disease from their recurrence.

Another very important point was evident from these trials—recurrences come late, 4 or more years after initial therapy. Other studies have shown that the average time for local recurrence is 9 or 10 years, much longer than is seen with infiltrating cancers. This is not surprising when we remember the basic concept of carcinomas in situ: the biopsies and treatments are occurring over a long, slow course of evolution from normal to cancerous, and that unless we completely eradicate the lesion, the course proceeds at its own rate.

Studies also have shown that the addition of *radiation therapy* impacts the course favorably. The recurrence rate was cut significantly, to 6% or 7%, but the local recurrences still occurred late. Why aren't the recurrences cut even more when radiation is added? In the initial therapy trials of cancer therapy that inadvertently included some patients with noninfiltrating cancers, it was noted by some researchers that patients who had extensive areas of intraductal cancer tended to do less well and had a higher local recurrence rate. In fact, in the early 1980s many radiotherapists were reluctant to treat patients with lumpectomy and radiation if their tumors had an extensive intraductal component.

Thanks to the work of Holland and his colleagues, we know the reason; intraductal cancers spread up and down the duct system, some extensively, and when the lumpectomies were being done, the margins were not clear. If the biopsy margins are truly negative, the local recurrence rates are lower.

Can All Intraductal Cancers Be Treated Conservatively?

Of course not. Many cancers, especially the cribriform type, are too extensive at presentation to permit breast conserving therapy and in others adequately clear margins cannot be achieved despite repeated excisions. In addition, some of the larger intraductal cancers actually have areas of microinvasion and a few of these actually spread to regional nodes.

It appears, therefore, that prognosis is determined to a great degree by size. This has been confirmed again and again, thanks to the studies of Lagios. He has demonstrated that the larger the tumor, the more likely that microinvasion exists. The cutoff seems to be at 25 mm. Other studies have shown that the larger the tumor, the more areas of microinvasion (which may or may not be evident initially), and the greater the chance of local nodal disease (large tumors begin to act like infiltrating cancers).

Although we know that noninfiltrating tumors vary in malignant appearance and in nuclear grade, and that some have hormone receptors and some express oncogene products, we have no idea how significant any of these factors are in their prognosis. From our knowledge of infiltrating cancers, we might presume that the more aggressive the tumor looks, the worse the prognosis for the patient, but we don't *know* that. Some intraductal cancers express oncogene products, such as Her-2-Neu, but no longer do so when they become infiltrating tumors. The significance of this is not known. At this time, these ancillary factors are not used in determining prognosis or therapy of carcinomas in situ.

Treatment

Intraductal cancers are treated as follows:

A *lesion under 10 mm* (Fig. 13-3), detected on mammography, and resected with clear, wide margins needs no further therapy. If the margin of the resection is involved with tumor, re-excision may be done. Search for metastases need not be done. A new baseline mammogram is obtained when healing is complete (before 6 months), and yearly thereafter. Careful examination by a physician should be done at 4-month intervals, remembering that recurrences appear late, averaging 8 to 10 years after diagnosis. Long-term survival, free of disease, should exceed 98%.

A *lesion 10 to 25 mm,* resected with *wide margins clear of tumor,* will probably benefit from postoperative radiotherapy. The chances of the axillary nodes being involved are so slight that no axillary sampling need be done. There is no need to search for metastases

Fig. 13-3. Treatment of intraductal cancers < 25 mm in size.

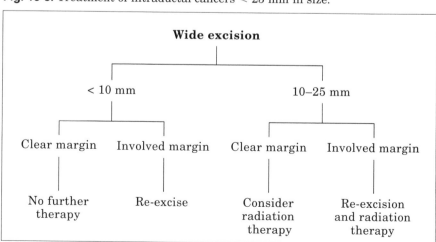

or to consider adjuvant therapy. Follow-up should be as discussed for lesions under 10 mm in size. Posttherapy baseline mammography should be obtained after radiation therapy is completed and the acute changes have subsided, which is usually in 2 to 3 months. Survival should exceed 98%.

A *lesion 10 to 25 mm,* in which the surgical margins are uncomfortably close (i.e., tumor within 1–2 mm of margin), even on repeat resection, should receive radiotherapy. Axillary dissection need not be done, nor is their a need to search for metastases. Follow-up is the same as discussed for lesions under 10 mm in size. Long-term survival, free of disease, should exceed 95%.

Lesions of 25 mm or greater should be treated as infiltrating cancer—with wide local resection and radiotherapy *or* total mastectomy (Fig. 13-4). If the margins are close after a local excision, reexcision may be considered in an attempt to obtain clear margins before radiotherapy. The feasibility of reexcision depends on the breast size and its advisability depends on the patient's desire for breast conservation.

The pathology must be reviewed carefully; if areas of microinvasion are seen, axillary dissection of the lowest level nodes may be warranted. The chance for metastatic disease is so small that no search need be made beyond routine chest x-ray and chemistry panel. If the axillary nodes are involved, the patient obviously had areas of invasion and adjuvant chemo- or hormonal therapy should

Fig. 13-4. Treatment of intraductal cancers > 25 mm in size.

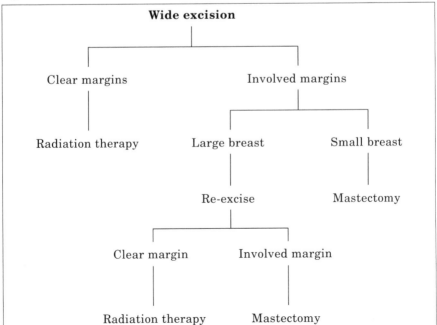

be considered. Currently, no one knows whether adjuvant therapy benefits patients with large intraductal cancers and negative axillary nodes. Follow-up should be similar to that for patients with infiltrating cancer (see Chap. 14). Survival should exceed 90%.

The chances of invasion increase directly with the size of the DCIS lesion. The risk of microinvasion for a 50-mm DCIS is approximately 50%. For that reason, some surgeons recommend axillary node dissection for these larger lesions, as they would for a known invasive cancer.

Suggested Reading

Risk

DuPont WD, and Page DL. Risk factors for breast cancer in women with proliferative breast disease. *N Engl J Med* 312:146–151, 1985.

DuPont WD, et al. Breast cancer risk associated with proliferative breast disease and atypical hyperplasia. *Cancer* 71:1258–1265, 1993.

Rosen PP. Proliferative breast "disease": An unresolved diagnostic dilemma. *Cancer* 71:3798–3807, 1993.

Diagnosis

Holland R, et al. Extent, distribution, and mammographic/histological correlations of breast ductal carcinoma in situ. *Lancet* 335:519–522, 1990.

Management

Fisher ER, et al. Conservative management of intraductal carcinoma (DCIS) of the breast. *J Surg Oncol* 47:139–147, 1991.

Fowble B. Intraductal noninvasive breast cancer: A comparison of three local treatments. Oncology 3:51–62, 1989.

Gallagher WJ, Koerner FC, and Wood WC. Treatment of intraductal carcinomas with limited surgery: Long-term follow-up. *J Clin Oncol* 7:376–380, 1989.

Ketcham AS, and Moffat FL. Vexed surgeons, perplexed patients, and breast cancers which may not be cancer. *Cancer* 65:387–393, 1990.

Lagios MD. Duct carcinoma in situ: Pathology and treatment. *Surg Clin North Am* 70:853–870, 1990.

Morrow M. Management of Nonpalpable Breast Lesions. Principles and Practice of Oncology (updates) 4:1–11, 1990.

Page DL, et al. Intraductal carcinoma of the breast: Follow-up after biopsy only. *Cancer* 49:751–758, 1982.

Recht A, et al. Therapy of in situ cancer. *Hematol Oncol Clin North Am* 3:691–708, 1989.

Solin LJ, et al. Ten-year results of breast-conserving surgery and definitive irradiation for intraductal carcinoma (ductal carcinoma in situ) of the breast. *Cancer* 68:2337–2344, 1991.

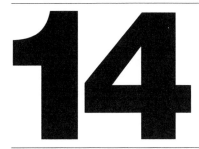

Invasive Breast Cancer: Staging and Treatment

Mary B. Rippon
and Janice K. Ryu

Today breast cancer is treated by a multidisciplinary team that includes surgeons, medical and radiation oncologists, and plastic surgeons. A woman newly diagnosed with breast cancer should be evaluated thoroughly to determine the clinical stage of her disease, and appropriate treatment options should be discussed. Several therapeutic choices may be available to her, especially if the cancer is in an early stage. This chapter will focus on the locoregional therapy of primary breast cancer. The roles of adjuvant chemotherapy and hormonal therapy will be discussed in Chap. 15.

Establishing the Diagnosis

The diagnosis of breast cancer can be made by several methods including fine needle aspiration (FNA), stereotoxic core biopsy, and open biopsy. These techniques are described in detail in Chap. 5.

The use of FNA to establish the diagnosis allows the physician to discuss treatment options with the patient before any surgery takes place. At the time of definitive surgery (i.e., mastectomy or lumpectomy and axillary node dissection), a frozen section often is performed because the FNA cannot distinguish between invasive and in situ (i.e., intraductal) carcinoma. This differentiation may alter the extent of the planned procedure. For example, an axillary node dissection is not required for in situ disease alone.

When an open surgical biopsy is done to establish the diagnosis, the potential for malignancy and the need for additional surgery should always be considered when determining the location of the biopsy incision. The biopsy specimen should be oriented for the pathologist and the margins inked to determine if all the tumor has been excised.

Clinical and Pathologic Staging

Staging System

Breast cancer is most commonly staged using the *TNM classification*. It is based on **T**umor size, palpable **N**odes, and **M**etastasis. This system is relatively easy to use and is outlined in Table 14-1. When reading the literature on breast cancer it is important to differentiate whether clinical or pathologic staging is being considered. The pathologic stage is determined after surgery when the actual tumor dimensions and the number of positive nodes are determined histologically. This stage can differ significantly from the clinical stage that is obtained on physical examination.

Recommended Tests

A few basic staging tests are recommended for all patients with a diagnosis of breast cancer, and others are reserved primarily for those who present with a more advanced stage (Table 14-2).

All breast cancer patients should have a *mammogram,* pref-

Table 14-1. TNM staging system

Definitions

Primary tumor (T)

X	Primary tumor cannot be assessed
T0	No evidence of primary tumor
Tis	Carcinoma in situ: intraductal carcinoma, lobular carcinoma in situ, Paget's disease without mass or invasion
T1	Tumor 2 cm or less in greatest dimension
T2	Tumor more than 2 cm but not more than 5 cm in greatest dimension
T3	Tumor more than 5 cm in greatest dimension
T4	Tumor of any size with direct extension to chest wall or skin; inflammatory carcinoma

Lymph node (N)

NX	Regional lymph nodes cannot be assessed (e.g., previously removed)
N0	No regional lymph node metastasis
N1	Metastasis to movable ipsilateral axillary lymph node(s)
N2	Metastasis to ipsilateral axillary lymph node(s) fixed to one another or to other structures
N3	Metastasis to ipsilateral internal mammary lymph node(s)

Distant metastasis (M)

MX	Presence of distant metastasis cannot be assessed
M0	No distant metastasis
M1	Distant metastasis (includes metastasis to ipsilateral supraclavicular lymph node[s])

Stage Grouping

Stage I	T1 N0 M0
Stage IIA	T0 N1 M0; T1 N1 M0; T2 N0 M0
Stage IIB	T2 N1 M0; T3 N0 M0
Stage IIIA	T0 N2 M0; T1 N2 M0; T2 N2 M0; T3 N1, N2 M0
Stage IIIB	T4 Any N M0; Any T N3 M0
Stage IV	Any T Any N M1

TNM = **T**umor size, palpable **N**odes, and **M**etastasis.
Source: Adapted from American Joint Committee on Cancer. *Manual for Staging of Cancer* (4th ed.). Philadelphia: Lippincott, 1992.

Table 14-2. Evaluation of the new breast cancer patient

Test	Breast cancer	
	Early (stage I and II)	Advanced (stage III and IV)
Mammogram	X	X
Liver function tests	X	X
Chext x-ray	X	X
Bone scan	If alkaline phosphatase levels increased or if patient symptomatic	X
Liver ultrasound or CT	If liver function tests abnormal	X
CA15-3*		X*

CT = computed tomography.
*Cancer antigen 15-3 (CA15-3) is considered investigational.

erably done before any diagnostic procedure is performed (i.e., FNA or biopsy). The mammogram is essential to rule out multifocal disease within the ipsilateral breast as well as contralateral breast disease. Determination of the extent of disease within the breast is of paramount importance for the discussion of reasonable treatment options with the patient. For example, a woman who appears to have multicentric disease or extensive suspicious microcalcifications throughout the breast is a poor candidate for breast conservation (Fig. 14-1).

Primary lab tests ordered are a *complete blood count* (CBC) and a full *chemistry panel* for all breast cancer patients. The chemistry panel provides basic screening for metastatic disease with liver function tests to screen for liver metastases, and alkaline phosphatase and calcium to screen for bone metastases. While these tests are not overly sensitive and do not completely rule out the possibility of metastases, they provide simple, cost-effective and adequate screening for women with early breast cancers. Finally a chest x-ray is ordered to screen for pulmonary metastases and to provide a baseline for later follow-up. If abnormalities are noted on any of these tests, more extensive and expensive tests are ordered to evaluate the abnormality.

Cancer antigen 15-3 (CA15-3) is a new serum marker for breast cancer that some oncologists include as one of the baseline tests for a woman diagnosed with breast cancer, in the hope that it can be an indicator of recurrent or metastatic disease. It does show some promise for use similar to carcinoembryonic antigen (CEA) in colon cancer. Like CEA it is not sensitive enough or cost-effective enough to be used as a screening test for breast cancer in the general population; CA15-3 levels will only be elevated in a very small percentage of patients with stage I or stage II breast cancer. Some oncologists have found CA15-3 helpful in correlating response to treatment for

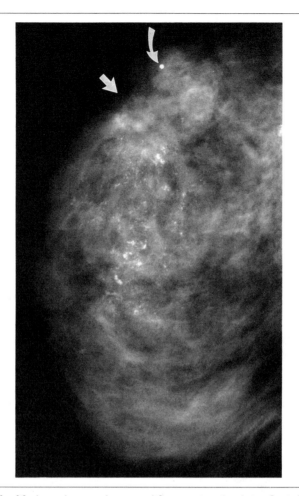

Fig. 14-1. Palpable invasive carcinoma with an extensive intraductal component (EIC). This right mediolateral mammogram shows an area of architectural distortion *(straight arrow)* that represents an invasive carcinoma. A radiopaque marker *(curved arrow)* had been placed on the patient's skin over the area of the palpable mass. In contiguity with the invasive cancer is a large area of malignant calcification inferiorly, which represents nonpalpable extensive intraductal tumor.

metastatic disease. At this point CA15-3 is still considered investigational and has not yet been approved by the FDA.

In women with early (stage I or II) breast cancer, further testing for metastatic disease in the absence of symptoms is neither indicated nor cost-effective. For example, approximately 1% of patients with stage I breast cancer have positive bone scans at presentation compared with 15% to 25% of stage III patients. For those women presenting with locally advanced cancers (i.e., tumors greater than 5 cm, peau d'orange or palpable nodes), additional staging studies should be considered to rule out metastatic disease. These additional tests include a bone scan and either an ultrasound or computed tomography (CT) of the liver.

As a screening test for hepatic metastases, *CT* is generally considered slightly more sensitive than ultrasound, especially for detecting smaller lesions. Liver ultrasound is less costly but more variable in quality because of its dependence on the expertise of the sonographer. If an inconclusive abnormality is detected on ultrasound, a liver CT scan can then be ordered to further evaluate the patient. Clinicians should be familiar with the expertise of their local radiologists when deciding which of these modalities to use in screening the liver for metastases. Scintigraphy lacks the resolution to image small lesions and is no longer used in screening for hepatic metastases. The use of magnetic resonance imaging (MRI) in hepatic screening is being investigated but is not yet as sensitive as CT, thus, the excess cost is not warranted.

For women presenting with locally advanced cancers, the chance of metastatic disease at presentation is considerably higher than in women with early stage (I and II) breast cancers, and its presence could significantly alter the treatment plan. More extensive screening with bone scan and hepatic imaging should be considered in these patients. Additional studies (e.g., bone scans) are also indicated in patients with symptoms such as hip or back pain that could represent metastatic disease.

Surgery for Breast Cancer

The surgical procedures performed for breast cancer are reviewed below.

Open Biopsy

Open biopsy is performed to establish the diagnosis of breast cancer and has been discussed in previous chapters. In most cases, an *excisional biopsy,* which attempts to remove the entire lesion, is done (see Chap. 5). If clear (i.e., negative) margins are obtained on the initial biopsy, the patient may be spared an additional procedure on the breast if the pathology is malignant. For a nonpalpable lesion, the assistance of the mammographer is required for needle localization (see Chap. 6).

An *incisional biopsy,* which removes only sufficient tumor to make the diagnosis, is done occasionally for large lesions prior to either mastectomy or induction chemotherapy.

The biopsy incision should be positioned so that it can later be incorporated into a lumpectomy or mastectomy in the event of a malignant diagnosis. A long tunnel between the incision site and the tumor should be avoided.

Lumpectomy

The term *lumpectomy* is used synonymously with wide excision, segmental mastectomy, and partial mastectomy. It signifies excision of the tumor with a negative margin (at least 1 cm) circumferentially. No drain is placed in the lumpectomy cavity because it is unnecessary in the vast majority of cases and can distort the contour of the breast. A seroma will initially fill the cavity and naturally remold the breast contour. The seroma fluid is gradually absorbed and replaced with scar tissue.

Axillary Node Dissection

Axillary node dissection is typically done in conjunction with a lumpectomy through a separate incision (Fig. 14-2) or as part of a mastectomy. The procedure is done to obtain valuable staging and prognostic information that may influence the treatment plan, even in the absence of clinically palpable lymph nodes. Approximately 40% of patients with invasive breast cancer will have involved nodes on pathologic examination of the surgical specimen that were often nonpalpable on clinical examination. Removal of the axillary nodes does *not* prevent the tumor from spreading to the nodes and is not done for that reason. It does, however, provide excellent local disease control in the axilla.

The level I and II lymph nodes should be included in a routine

Fig. 14-2. Illustration of the separate incisions used for lumpectomy and axillary node dissection. Location of the breast incision will vary with tumor location. (Adapted from Kinne, DW. Surgery. In JR Harris et al, Breast Diseases [2nd ed]. Philadelphia: Lippincott, 1991.)

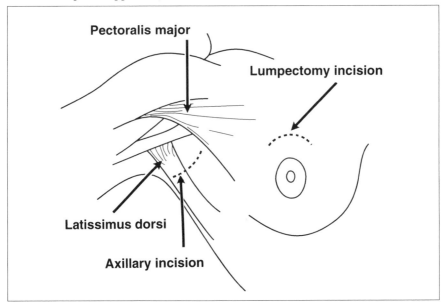

axillary dissection. Anatomically these are the nodes that lie lateral to (level I) and underneath (level II) the pectoralis minor muscle. Removal of the muscle is not necessary to obtain the nodes. When the level I and II nodes are negative, the chances are miniscule (1–2%) that the highest level III nodes, medial to the pectoralis minor muscle, will be involved; thus their routine removal is not required. Omitting the level III nodes may slightly decrease the risk of arm edema, especially in the patient who subsequently receives radiation to the axilla. Grossly involved nodes at all levels should always be removed at the time of surgery. A surgical drain is placed in the axilla prior to closing the incision and usually remains in place 5 to 10 days postoperatively to prevent the accumulation of blood and lymphatic fluid.

An axillary node "sampling" instead of a formal anatomic axillary dissection involves removing a few superficial lymph nodes that are usually attached to the axillary tail of the breast. Although sampling may be faster, it often provides inadequate information and is not recommended. For example, if only five nodes are obtained in the sample and they are found to be negative, is it then safe to assume that the patient is "node-negative" when the axilla potentially contains 20 to 40 lymph nodes? An axillary dissection should provide a minimum of 10 to 12 lymph nodes for pathologic examination. A formal anatomic dissection also provides a measure of consistency between different institutions and surgeons when comparing treatment outcomes.

For the patient who has pure in situ disease, without any evidence of invasion, axillary dissection is not required because the incidence of nodal involvement is less than 1%.

Mastectomy

Simple mastectomy removes the breast alone and does not include an axillary node dissection. This procedure may be used for the treatment of in situ disease or in the patient undergoing prophylactic mastectomy in whom nodal involvement is not expected.

The most common procedure used in the treatment of breast cancer has been *modified radical mastectomy*. With this procedure, the breast and axillary nodes are removed in continuity. Axillary node dissection is an inherent part of a modified radical mastectomy and thus is not specified separately as when done in conjunction with lumpectomy. The incision usually runs obliquely from near the sternum to the axilla, and the pectoralis muscles are not removed.

Radical mastectomy is included for reasons of completeness and historical interest. Current indications for this procedure are almost nonexistent. The procedure includes a modified radical mastectomy with the additional removal of the pectoralis major and minor muscles. Because this basically leaves only the ribs on the chest wall, the patient is left with a flat, almost scaphoid appearance. Until modified radical mastectomy was proved equally effective, radical mastectomy was the procedure of choice for breast cancer. Now it is reserved for patients who have extensive involvement of the entire pectoralis major or both major and minor muscles. Local fixation or focal involvement of the muscle can be addressed by resecting only the involved portion of the muscle.

The length of surgery and hospital stay are similar for patients undergoing modified radical mastectomy and those who have a lumpectomy and axillary node dissection. Both procedures are routinely performed under general anesthesia, and the vast majority of women (of all ages) are discharged home within 24 to 48 hours of their surgery. At the time of discharge the drain(s) remain in place. The patient is instructed to empty the drain(s) and record the output on a daily basis. The drains are removed in approximately 5 to 10 days depending on the amount of output.

Treatment Options for Early Breast Cancer (Stage I and II)

The woman who presents with an early breast cancer usually has several surgical options. The primary decision to be made is between modified radical mastectomy (i.e., removal of the entire breast and the axillary nodes) and breast conservation. The presence of palpable nodes in the axilla is not a contraindication to breast preservation. With mastectomy, immediate or delayed reconstruction may be considered.

Breast Conservation

Breast conservation therapy for invasive breast cancer consists of lumpectomy and axillary node dissection followed by radiation therapy to treat the remainder of the breast. For most women this is appealing because the surgery is perceived to be less mutilating and allows them to maintain their natural breast tissue and contour. It is important for the patient and her clinicians to realize that *the survival rate is the same whether she chooses breast conservation or modified radical mastectomy.*

Several large prospective randomized studies from the United States and Europe indicate that lumpectomy and axillary node dissection followed by whole breast irradiation are equivalent to mastectomy in the management of early stage breast cancer. When appropriate selection criteria are applied, the locoregional recurrence rate with breast conservation therapy should be in the range of 5% to 10% at 5 years (Table 14-3). Disease-free and overall survival are dependent primarily on nodal involvement and tumor size.

The B-06 trial conducted by the National Surgical Adjuvant Breast and Bowel Project (NSABP) was one of the largest trials comparing the efficacy of breast conservation to the standard mastectomy.

Table 14-3. Locoregional recurrence and survival
after breast conservation therapy

Institution	Locoregional recurrence (%)		Surviving at 10 years, by stage (%)		
	5 years	10 years	I	II	I and II
Joint Center for Radiation Therapy	10	16	85	57	
University of Pennsylvania	8	18	87	77	
NSABP	8	10*	83*	68*	
Institut Gustave-Roussy	7	10			78
Italian National Cancer Institute (Milan)		6			75

NSABP = National Surgical Adjuvant Breast Project.
*8-year results.

Patients were enrolled in this study from 1976 to 1984, so that there is now more than 8 years of follow-up. Patients were randomized to one of three treatment groups: (1) modified radical mastectomy, (2) lumpectomy with axillary node dissection, or (3) lumpectomy with axillary node dissection followed by whole breast irradiation. Nearly 2000 women with tumors less than 4 cm and histologically negative margins obtained at the time of surgery comprised the study population. Both node-negative and node-positive patients were included with the node-positive patients also receiving systemic chemotherapy. The most recent study update, with an 8-year follow-up, showed no significant difference in survival between the three treatment groups. However, those that underwent lumpectomy and node dissection *without* breast irradiation experienced a significant increase in local recurrence compared with the other two groups (40% vs. 10–15%). Thus, radiation therapy is considered an integral part of breast conservation as a treatment option.

Several ongoing studies are attempting to identify subgroups of patients that may have a very low rate of local recurrence even without radiation therapy. Until further data are available to identify favorable subgroups, breast preservation without radiation therapy should be offered to patients only in the setting of clinical trials. Adjuvant chemotherapy should be considered as systemic therapy, which is relatively ineffective in controlling local disease and should not be viewed as an alternative to breast irradiation.

Patient Selection
Breast conservation is a viable option for the majority of women who present with early breast cancer but certain patient- and tumor-related factors make some patients poor candidates for this form of treatment (Table 14-4).

Table 14-4. Eligibility for breast conservation

Good candidate	Marginal candidate	Poor candidate
Tumors < 4–5 cm in size	Tumors > 5 cm in diameter (T3 lesions)	Gross multifocal or multicentric disease
Average breast size	Extensive intraductal component in presence of invasive tumor	Diffuse microcalcification on mammogram
Negative or focally positive microscopic margin of resection		Grossly positive surgical margin
Reliable patient		Severe collagen vascular disease
		Noncompliant patient for daily radiation therapy
		Pregnant woman
		Previous radiation therapy to partial or whole breast

TUMOR-RELATED FACTORS. Consideration for breast conservation requires that the breast size be adequate in proportion to the *tumor size* to allow complete resection with a good cosmetic result. A tumor size of 5 cm is an arbitrary cutoff chosen by many to be the upper limit for breast conserving therapy. This is based in part on the difficulty of preserving adequate breast tissue to obtain an acceptable cosmetic result in the average-sized breast after resecting the large tumor with a margin of normal tissue. This, however, may be quite feasible in the large-breasted woman. There have been reports that indicate an increased risk of subclinical multicentricity with tumors greater than 5 cm (T3 lesions). One of the goals of radiation therapy is to eradicate subclinical microscopic disease that may be present in the remaining breast tissue; however, it is possible that the medium-dose irradiation routinely used may not eradicate extensive multifocal disease that may be associated with large lesions. Patients with large tumors have a significantly increased risk for distant metastatic disease, which is more likely to determine their overall survival. Therefore, although previous clinical trials of breast conservation excluded women with tumors greater than 4 to 5 cm, studies are currently under way to evaluate the outcome of breast conserving surgery and radiation in this group of patients. It is critical that the tumor size always be evaluated in relation to breast size when determining patient eligibility for breast conservation.

Location of the tumor in the subareolar region is not a contraindication to breast conservation but does require removal by central lumpectomy of the nipple-areolar complex. Some patients find this cosmetically unacceptable and elect to have a mastectomy. Other women are pleased to maintain their breast mound and contour despite the loss of the nipple. The nipple-areolar complex can later be reconstructed if the patient so desires.

Clinical evidence of gross multicentric disease extending beyond one quadrant, either on physical examination or mammogram, is an absolute contraindication to breast conservation. Multifocality within a single quadrant of the breast can be encompassed with a quadrantectomy (a more extensive lumpectomy that has been done routinely in some European centers). A patient with tumors in two totally separate areas of the breast demonstrated by biopsy or FNA to be malignant, or with diffuse suspicious microcalcifications, would not be a good candidate for breast conservation and modified radical mastectomy is recommended.

Invasive tumor at a surgical margin (i.e., a "positive margin") or the presence of an extensive intraductal component (EIC) are tumor-related factors considered to be relative contraindications for breast conservation.

The precise definition of *EIC* is controversial in the literature, and different pathologists may use different criteria. One of the most commonly used definitions for EIC, provided by Holland and his colleagues at the Harvard Joint Center for Radiation Therapy, is an invasive tumor with an intraductal component that comprises 25% or more of the primary tumor *and* is present at the margin of resection in the surrounding normal breast tissue. The presence of these features in a specimen is associated with a higher recurrence rate in the breast (25–30%). In most cases, re-excision is recommended to achieve negative microscopic margins. If re-excision continues to reveal involvement of the margin with invasive or intraductal carcinoma, a mastectomy should be performed. In cases in which a margin is focally positive (i.e., a single focus), in the absence of EIC, re-excision of that margin can be done if cosmetically feasible; otherwise the patient can proceed directly to radiation therapy.

Factors *not* associated with an increased recurrence rate in the breast after breast conservation are axillary node status, tumor location, tumor size up to 5 cm, lobular histology, and a microscopically positive margin of resection at a single focus. The presence of positive axillary nodes either on physical examination or at the time of surgery is *not* a contraindication to breast preserving surgery.

PATIENT-RELATED FACTORS. Patient-related factors that make breast conservation a poor therapeutic option include those medical conditions that rule out delivery of breast irradiation with acceptable side effects and cosmetic results. Patients with a history of severe collagen vascular disorders have an increased risk of subcutaneous fibrosis, necrosis, and telangiectasias. Pregnant women should not receive radiation therapy to the breast because of the potential scatter to the fetus that can occur despite abdominal shielding. Patients who have received prior irradiation to the area of the involved breast, such as for Hodgkin's disease or thyroid disease, should not be offered breast conservation if additional radiation cannot be safely delivered to the breast.

Large breast size and *obesity* have been considered relative contraindications to breast conservation. Several studies of radiation therapy in this group of patients have shown less than optimal cosmetic results due to increased telangiectasias, persistent edema, retraction, and fibrosis. Greater acute skin reaction and edema has been observed during and immediately after radiation therapy. One factor contributing to these poor results in these patients is dose inhomogeneity within the breast that causes "hot" spots in substantial portions of the breast. The use of higher energy photons and meticulous technique may circumvent poor dose distribution and provide a better cosmetic result. Thus, obesity or large breast size should not exclude patients from consideration for breast conservation. One needs to remember that these same women would have marked asymmetry with mastectomy and may have difficulty with reconstruction as well.

Young age has been implicated as a risk factor for increased breast recurrence after conservative surgery and radiation. This is currently a controversial topic and more data are needed to determine whether in fact young age is a poor prognostic factor for local recurrence, independent of other histopathologic features. Thus, patient age (at this time) should not be a reason to render patients ineligible for breast conservation therapy.

From a psychosocial standpoint the patient who opts for breast conservation has to be willing to come for daily visits, Monday through Friday, for 5 to 6 weeks, to complete the radiation component. Therefore, breast conservation is not a good option for the patient who cannot or will not comply.

Any woman who is a potential candidate for breast conservation should be encouraged to consult with a radiation oncologist before her definitive surgery to fully explore what is involved with the radiation therapy. It also provides the opportunity for the radiation oncologist to determine whether the patient is an appropriate candidate for radiation therapy and whether a good cosmetic result can be anticipated.

Breast Irradiation

One of the most important determinants of the overall cosmetic result and of both acute and late complications of breast conservation therapy is the technique of breast irradiation. Planning radiation therapy involves careful review and integration of clinical, radiographic, and pathologic information, including the size and location of the primary tumor, the status of the axillary lymph nodes, and the surgical margins. The amount of possible residual tumor burden in the breast and the risk of regional lymphatic involvement are estimated and used to determine the dose to the whole breast, the boost to the primary tumor bed, and whether to treat the regional lymphatics.

Prior to the initiation of radiation therapy, every patient participates in a radiation planning session, or "simulation," which lasts approximately 1½ hours. During simulation, the patient is placed in the treatment position with her arm raised above her head while a cast of her upper torso, including her raised arm and shoulder, is made in this position (Fig. 14-3). The cast is made so that the daily set-up position can be reproduced with minimal variability. Tiny tattoos are placed on the anterior and lateral chest wall for the same purpose. These tattoos, although permanent, resemble a freckle and generally do not cause the patient any concern.

Simulation usually occurs 3 to 5 weeks after definitive surgery to allow the adequate healing and return of shoulder mobility that is required to maintain the treatment position. Daily radiation therapy then begins 5 days a week for approximately 6 to 6½ weeks. Each treatment lasts approximately 15 minutes and delivers 180 to 200 cGy (rads). First, the whole breast is irradiated and then a boost is given to the primary tumor bed. The standard dose of radiation to the breast is 4500 to 5000 cGy. The axilla is not included in the radiation field if an adequate axillary dissection reveals pathologically negative lymph nodes or if the primary tumor consists of only in situ disease.

Indications for irradiation of the axilla vary from institution to institution because the axilla is technically treated with surgery and recurrence in the axilla is uncommon after an adequate axillary dissection. The risk of axillary recurrence is increased, however, with involvement of multiple lymph nodes, extracapsular extension of tumor outside the lymph nodes, or extensive matting of the lymph nodes. If axillary recurrence does occur, it is often difficult to eradicate with radiation or surgery and can cause significant local morbidity. Patients at high risk for axillary recurrence should receive an additional boost from the posterior axilla to complement the dose delivered from the anterior field. Some institutions routinely deliver radiation to the axilla if the number of involved axillary nodes

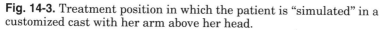

Fig. 14-3. Treatment position in which the patient is "simulated" in a customized cast with her arm above her head.

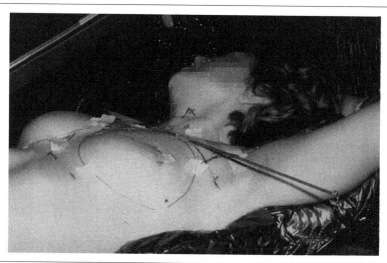

exceeds three, while other centers will individualize on a case by case basis weighing the extent of surgery as well as the risk of axillary recurrence and arm edema.

Indications for radiation treatment of the supraclavicular fossa include multiple, pathologically positive axillary lymph nodes, no axillary dissection, or an inadequate axillary lymph node dissection (e.g., an axillary sampling). Approximately one-third of patients with positive axillary nodes have microscopic metastases to the supraclavicular lymph nodes. The treatment of the supraclavicular fossa adds minimal morbidity; thus, most patients with positive axillary lymph nodes should have the supraclavicular fossa included in the radiation field.

The prophylactic treatment of the internal mammary nodes (IMN) is even more controversial. Although histopathologic studies have demonstrated significant risk of IMN metastases in patients with axillary nodal involvement, especially with tumors in the medial quadrants of the breast, the clinical appearance of IMN recurrence is rare (2–3%), and the impact of IMN irradiation on overall survival is unclear. In addition, the treatment of the IMN chain is technically challenging if all lymph nodes are to be treated while at the same time dose delivery to normal tissues such as heart and lung is minimized. Therefore, IMN radiation is not generally employed.

Patients should be informed that chemotherapy does not interfere with the delivery of breast irradiation when correctly sequenced with the appropriate chemotherapeutic agents. The sequencing of chemotherapy and radiation therapy varies among major cancer centers and is the subject of several current studies.

Complications of Radiation Therapy

Definitive breast irradiation is well tolerated and associated with minimal long-term complications. *Rib fracture* occurs in less than 5% of patients; older patients with preexisting osteoporosis may be at a slightly increased risk for this complication. Radiation-induced rib fractures rarely pose a clinical problem and heal without intervention.

If optimal radiation techniques are employed that minimize the amount of lung tissue exposed, the incidence of symptomatic *radiation pneumonitis* should also be less than 5%. The symptoms of radiation pneumonitis include dry cough, shortness of breath, and a low-grade fever. The diagnosis is made when the chest radiograph demonstrates an interstitial pattern of infiltrates on the treated side, which in the case of breast irradiation corresponds to the peripheral lung fields. Other causes of pneumonitis, including infection or lymphangitic spread of tumor, must be excluded before a diagnosis of radiation pneumonitis is made. Most cases of radiation pneumonitis are self-limited and do not require intervention. A short course of steroids may be helpful in severe cases to resolve symptoms.

The risk of severe *arm edema* is increased when the axillary bed has been fully irradiated, especially after an axillary dissection that included level III (highest) lymph nodes. The patient body mass appears to be an important risk factor for arm edema, thus obesity increases risk.

The *carcinogenic potential* of radiation, either as an incidental exposure or as a treatment for malignancy, has been a topic of great interest and concern. It has been established that a linear increase in the risk of carcinogenesis occurs at low doses of radiation exposure, but it appears the risk is negligible at therapeutic doses. The risk of radiation-induced breast cancer is increased when the low-dose radiation is experienced during the early teenage years when the breast tissue develops. Fortunately, most breast cancer patients are over the age of 30. The opposite breast receives a scatter dose of radiation in the range of 100 to 200 cGy over the course of usual breast irradiation. The risk of contralateral breast cancer induction in patients undergoing breast conserving treatment has been extensively studied. Contralateral breast cancer represents up to 50% of second malignancies in breast cancer patients. However, most studies of contralateral breast cancer in patients undergoing lumpectomy and radiation yield risks similar to those observed in mastectomy series.

There are sporadic reports of sarcoma, leukemia, and possibly lung cancer after radiation therapy of the breast or chest wall. Solid tumors (i.e., sarcoma, lung cancer) tend to appear after a latency period of 10 to 18 years. Based on data from the Connecticut Breast Cancer Registry, Kurtz and colleagues estimated that in every 1000 women surviving 5 years or more after treatment, two radiation-induced soft tissue sarcomas will occur per each decade of follow-up. According to Fowble and colleagues, this represents a smaller risk than that which exists for lymphangiosarcoma arising in the edematous arm and shoulder in women that underwent radical mastectomy. Most studies find no correlation between breast or chest wall irradiation and leukemia. The NSABP B-06 and Milan studies indicate essentially the same risk of secondary nonbreast solid malignancies for patients undergoing mastectomy (2%) and for those treated with lumpectomy and radiation therapy (2–3%). Concern about the risk of secondary malignancy should not, therefore, be a deterrent to the patient considering radiation therapy as part of her treatment plan.

Cosmetic Results

The second goal of breast-preserving therapy, after disease eradication, is to attain the best cosmetic result possible given the confines of the tumor and any other patient-related factors that might exist. Clearly any evaluation of cosmetic result is quite subjective, and the opinions of the patient and her different health practitioners may differ. The scale shown in Table 14-5 was initially developed by Harris and colleagues and is frequently used in the oncologic community

Table 14-5. Cosmetic rating after lumpectomy and breast irradiation

Excellent	Treated breast almost identical to untreated breast
Good	Slight difference between treated and untreated breast
Fair	Obvious difference between treated and untreated breast
Poor	Marked distortion of the treated breast

Source: Adapted from Harris JR, et al. Analysis of cosmetic results following primary radiation for Stages I and II carcinoma of the breast. *Int J Radiat Oncol Biol Phys* 5: 257, 1979.

to assess the cosmetic result after conservative surgery and radiation.

Most of the series that have evaluated breast preserving surgery followed by radiation therapy report good to excellent results in 70% to 90% of patients treated. Examples of different cosmetic results after lumpectomy and radiation therapy are illustrated in Figs. 14-4 and 14-5. One of the most important determinants of cosmetic result is the extent and technique of surgical resection. The extent of resection determines the amount of tissue defect and potential asymmetry but this is at least partly determined by the tumor size. The location and type of incision also contributes to the overall cosmetic result. The extent of axillary dissection may be associated with breast edema as well as arm edema. Radiation therapy determinants for cosmetic result include total dose delivered, daily fraction size, boost technique and volume, poor matchline technique, and concurrent use of Adriamycin or methotrexate chemotherapy regimens.

Modified Radical Mastectomy

Modified radical mastectomy is a standard option in the treatment of breast cancer. It must be remembered, however, that for many, if not most, patients *it is not the only option*. It is the procedure of choice in patients who are not candidates for breast conservation for one or more of the reasons noted in the preceding sections.

Postmastectomy Breast Irradiation

Tremendous controversy surrounds the use of postmastectomy chest wall irradiation for prophylaxis against the locoregional recurrence of breast cancer. Early prospective randomized trials conducted in the United States by NSABP (B-02 trial) and in Europe (Stockholm, Manchester, Oslo trials) demonstrated no survival benefit when mastectomy and postoperative chest wall irradiation was compared to mastectomy alone despite the universal finding of decreased locoregional failure with adjuvant radiation therapy. These trials have been criticized, however, for poor radiation technique and inadequate radiation dose, inclusion of patients at low risk for locoregional failure, and lack of stratification by prognostic factors.

Previous epidemiologic studies of long-term (15-year) survival

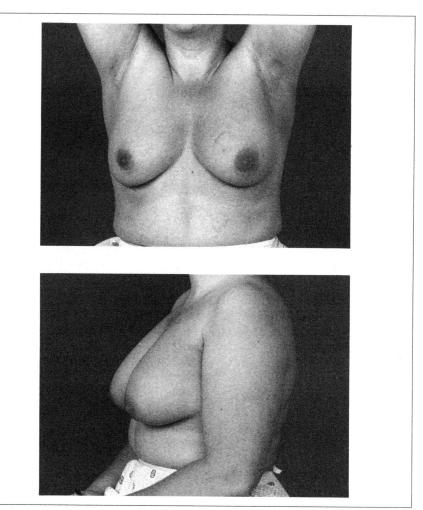

Fig. 14-4. Good cosmetic result in a patient who has undergone lumpectomy, axillary node dissection, and radiation therapy on the left side. Note the symmetry of the breasts and lack of discoloration or retraction in the treated breast.

rates of the patients randomized in these studies have hinted at increased late cardiovascular deaths in those who had received post-mastectomy radiation therapy. Radiation therapy techniques have evolved since the time these studies were conducted and a significant dose is no longer delivered to the heart or the coronary arteries.

It is still important to apply postmastectomy radiation therapy judiciously for those patients at high risk for locoregional recurrence. High-risk patients include those with tumors 5 cm or larger, chest wall or gross skin involvement with tumor, diffuse lymphatic invasion within the breast or dermis, positive margins on the mastectomy specimen, or four or more positive lymph nodes. For each of these indications the risk of locoregional recurrence is estimated to be 25%

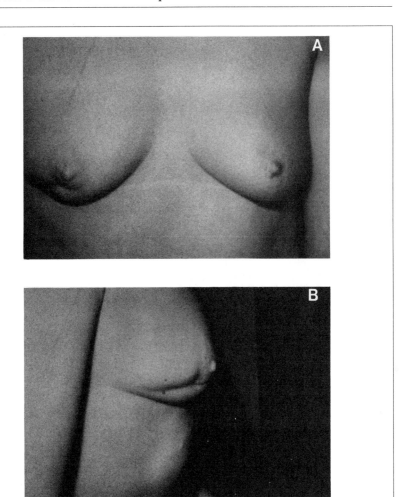

Fig. 14-5. Poor cosmetic results after breast conserving therapy. Frontal (A) and lateral (B) views of a patient with significant scar retraction after conservative surgery and radiation therapy. C. Marked telangiectasia after radiation therapy resulted in a poor cosmetic result. D. Note the size discrepancy of the treated breast *(left)*, a suboptimal cosmetic result.

to 30%. Postoperative radiation therapy can reduce locoregional recurrence in this high-risk group to less than 10%.

The field for postoperative radiation therapy includes the chest wall and supraclavicular fossa. When multiple matted or fixed nodes (N_2 disease) or extension into soft tissue outside the nodes is reported, the posterior axilla is boosted. The standard dose for postmastectomy radiation therapy is approximately 5000 cGy over 5 to 5½ weeks with a technique similar to that used with breast conservation.

Postmastectomy radiation therapy can cause more erythema and desquamation of the skin compared to irradiation of an intact breast. The chest wall skin receives almost full-dose treatment because it is

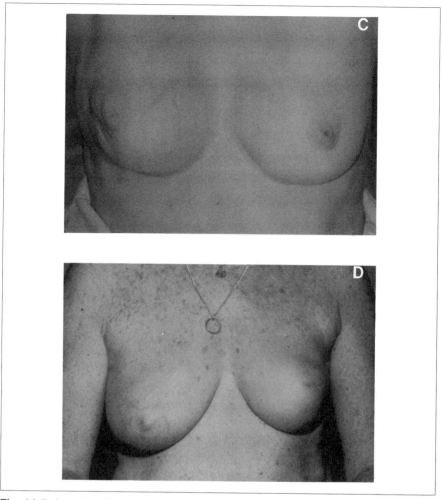

Fig. 14-5. (continued)

one of the target tissues for postoperative treatment, while the skin over an intact breast is spared to a greater degree when irradiated. Otherwise, the complications associated with postmastectomy breast irradiation are the same as those described for conservative therapy.

Modified Radical Mastectomy with Reconstruction

With modified radical mastectomy with reconstruction, the patient may have several additional choices to make, the first being immediate (i.e., at the time of definitive resection) versus delayed reconstruction. The advantage of the immediate approach is that the patient wakes up with "something there," rather than feeling flat. This in some ways diminishes the loss and may also eliminate at least one additional surgery. On the other hand, delayed reconstruction provides the patient with more time to reach a decision on the type of reconstruction (if any) that she wants, rather than trying to make that decision amidst all the emotions experienced by one newly diagnosed with breast cancer. Delayed reconstruction also may be advantageous to the patient who will require additional therapy in the form of radiation therapy or chemotherapy. Immediate reconstruction potentially could delay adjuvant chemotherapy or radiation therapy if problems occur with wound healing. If a tissue expander is placed, postmastectomy radiation therapy (if indicated) usually is delayed until the expansion is complete.

Several options for reconstruction are available, such as implants and various tissue flaps. Interested patients should be advised to consult with a plastic surgeon to explore these possibilities. A more thorough discussion of reconstruction can be found in Chap. 20.

Radiation Therapy After Breast Reconstruction

Radiation therapy can be delivered safely to the augmented or reconstructed breast—in the patient with a tissue flap or an implant. Silicone has been shown to be "tissue-equivalent," and radiation has similar depth distribution in both silicone and breast tissue. If a tissue expander was placed in the breast by the surgeon at the time of mastectomy and the patient requires postoperative radiation, we delay radiation until the expansion is completed but prior to the placement of the permanent implant. Because many of these patients also require chemotherapy, this can be given concomitantly with the tissue expansion and the radiation following. Radiation therapy of silicone implants has been associated with a slightly increased risk for capsular contracture. Such contractures occur more frequently when radiation is administered soon after placement of the silicone implant. There is also some evidence that subcutaneous and subglandular implants are more likely to develop encapsulation after radiation therapy than are submuscular implants. If a patient develops a painful or cosmetically deforming capsular contracture after radiation therapy, the patient has the option of revision encapsulectomy and placement of another implant. If it is anticipated preoperatively that a patient will require postmastectomy radiation (e.g., tumor > 5 cm, multiple palpable or matted nodes) then the patient may be better served by a delayed rather than an immediate reconstruction. Irradiated chest wall skin can be expanded for delayed reconstruction later. The risk of wound breakdown due to previous radiation therapy is low when the patient is in the hands of an experienced reconstructive surgeon.

Treatment of Locally Advanced Breast Cancer

Included in this group are patients who present with large tumors (e.g., >5 cm), large or matted nodes, skin involvement, or peau d'orange. Generally they are not good candidates for breast conservation because the extent of the primary breast tumor or matted, fixed adenopathy is not well encompassed with a lumpectomy and node dissection. These patients are usually treated with all three modalities—surgery, chemotherapy, and radiation therapy—to optimize their disease-free and overall survival. Many oncologists advocate preoperative chemotherapy to shrink the tumor, to enhance the potential of obtaining clear margins, to test the drug responsiveness of the tumor, and to address microscopic systemic disease early. Others proceed directly with mastectomy if the tumor is resectable.

If preoperative chemotherapy decreases the tumor size sufficiently, lumpectomy followed by radiation therapy may be considered. Breast conservation for locally advanced tumors is being investigated at several institutions in this country and in Italy but is not yet considered standard therapy. It is more common practice to perform a mastectomy even with significant tumor shrinkage.

For tumors considered unresectable because of size, extent of skin involvement, or fixation to the chest wall, induction chemotherapy should be administered to attempt to make the tumor resectable without an extensive skin or chest wall resection and reconstruction. Chemotherapy may be followed by preoperative radiation therapy in an attempt to improve the resectability of the tumor. Occasionally, chemotherapy and radiation are given concurrently in an attempt to make refractory tumors resectable. Additional cycles of chemotherapy are also given postoperatively.

Inflammatory Breast Cancer

This is a relatively rare presentation of breast cancer. As the name implies, the patient presents with rapid onset of an erythematous, hot, and sometimes tender breast. Frequently mistaken for mastitis, the patient is often placed on antibiotics. Mastitis is certainly more common than inflammatory breast cancer, but the clinician should be suspicious if the symptoms do not resolve with a short course of antibiotics or if they occur in women unlikely to be at risk for mastitis (e.g., a postmenopausal, nonlactating female). A palpable mass may not be apparent. A biopsy of the inflamed skin, which represents the presence of dermal lymphatic invasion by tumor, generally provides the diagnosis.

Chemotherapy should be the primary treatment modality. Inflammatory carcinoma represents a very aggressive tumor with a high risk of systemic spread, thus chemotherapy needs to begin as soon as possible. Response to this induction chemotherapy is indicated by resolution of the erythema or a decrease in size of any palpable mass. After the cycles of induction chemotherapy are completed, locoregional therapy is initiated. Although the sequence may vary based on institutional preference, both surgery (modified radical mastectomy) and radiation therapy are employed in most cases. There is no significant advantage to either sequence of local therapy, with respect to either locoregional recurrence or survival. Some tumors necessitate radiation therapy first in order to make them resectable. Additional systemic chemotherapy is administered after the locoregional therapy is completed.

In the past, 5-year survival for this inflammatory breast cancer was zero but the survival rate has improved significantly, to 30%, with an aggressive combined modality approach utilizing chemotherapy, surgery, and radiation therapy. Chest wall and regional lymphatic radiation is essential in the management of both locally advanced and inflammatory carcinomas. Tamoxifen may also be given when other therapies are concluded.

The role of adjuvant chemotherapy and hormonal therapy is discussed in a comprehensive fashion in Chap. 15. Guidelines for appropriate follow-up of the patient with breast cancer are presented in Chap. 19.

Suggested Reading

General

Fowble B. Local-Regional Treatment Options for Early Invasive Breast Cancer. In B Fowble et al. (eds). *Breast Cancer Treatment: A Comprehensive Guide to Management.* St. Louis: Mosby–Year Book, 1991. Pp. 25–88.

Fowble B. The Role of Postmastectomy Adjuvant Radiotherapy for Operable Breast Cancer. In B Fowble et al. (eds). *Breast Cancer Treatment: A Comprehensive Guide to Management.* St. Louis: Mosby–Year Book, 1991. Pp. 289–310.

Fowble B, Solin L, and Schultz D. Conservative Surgery and Radiation for Early Breast Cancer. In B Fowble et al. (eds). *Breast Cancer Treatment: A Comprehensive Guide to Management.* St. Louis: Mosby–Year Book, 1991. Pp. 105–150.

Kinne D. Primary Treatment of Breast Cancer. In J Harris, et al. (eds). *Breast Disease* (2nd ed.). Philadelphia: Lippincott, 1991. Pp. 347–372.

Staging Studies for Breast Cancer

American Joint Committee on Cancer. *Manual for Staging of Cancer* (4th ed.). Philadelphia: Lippincott, 1992.

McNeil B, Pace PD, and Gray E. Pre-operative and follow-up bone scans in patients with primary carcinoma of the breast. *Surg Gynecol Obstet* 147:745–748, 1978.

Wernecke R, et al. Detection of hepatic masses in patients with carcinoma: Comparative sensitivities of sonography, CT and MR imaging. *AJR* 157:731, 1991.

Breast Conservation in Early Breast Cancer

Fisher B, et al. Five year results of a randomized clinical trial comparing total mastectomy and segmental mastectomy with or without radiation in the treatment of breast cancer. *N Engl J Med* 312:665, 1985.

Fisher B, et al. Eight-year results of a randomized clinical trial comparing total mastectomy and lumpectomy with or without irradiation in the treatment of breast cancer. *N Engl J Med* 320:822, 1989.

Harris JL, et al. Analysis of cosmetic results following primary radiation for Stages I and II carcinoma of the breast. *Int J Radiat Oncol Biol Phys* 5:257, 1979.

Holland R, et al. The presence of an extensive intraductal component following a limited excision correlates with prominent residual disease in the remainder of the breast. *J Clin Oncol* 8:113, 1990.

Recht A, and Harris JR. Selection of patients with early-stage breast cancer for conservative surgery and radiation. *Oncology* 4:23, 1990.

Veronesi U. Breast Conservation Trials of the NCI Milan. In Proceedings of the NIH Consensus Development Conference—Early Stage Breast Cancer, June 19, 1990. Pp. 19–22.

Locally Advanced Breast Cancer

Bonadonna G, et al. Primary chemotherapy to avoid mastectomy in tumors with diameters of three centimeters or more. *J Natl Cancer Inst* 82:1539, 1990.

Jacquillat MD, et al. Results of neoadjuvant chemotherapy and radiation therapy in the breast-conserving treatment of 250 patients with all stages of infiltrative breast cancer. *Cancer* 66:119, 1990.

Jaeyesimi IA, Buzdar AU, and Hortobagyi G. Inflammatory breast cancer: A review. *J Clin Oncol* 10:1014, 1992.

Singletary SE, McNeese MD, and Hortobagyi N. Feasibility of breast-conservation surgery after induction chemotherapy for locally advanced breast carcinoma. *Cancer* 69:2849, 1992.

Postmastectomy Breast Irradiation

Fowble B, Glick J, and Goodman R. Radiotherapy for the prevention of local-regional recurrence in high risk patients post mastectomy receiving adjuvant chemotherapy. *Int J Radiat Oncol Biol Phys* 15: 627–631, 1988.

Complications of Radiation Therapy

Cuzick J, et al. Overview of randomized trials of postoperative adjuvant radiotherapy in breast cancer. *Cancer Treat Res* 71:15, 1987.

Fowble B. Local-Regional Treatment Options for Early Invasive Breast Cancer. In B Fowble, et al. (eds). *Breast Cancer Treatment: A Comprehensive Guide to Management.* St. Louis: Mosby–Year Book, 1991. Pp. 64–66.

Jones JM, and Ribeiro GG. Mortality patterns over 34 years of breast cancer patients in a clinical trial of post-operative radiotherapy. *Clin Radiol* 40:204, 1989.

Kurtz JM, et al. Contralateral breast cancer and other second malignancies in patients treated by breast conserving therapy with radiation. *Int J Radiat Oncol Biol Phys* 15:277, 1988.

Larson P, et al. Edema of the arm as a function of the extent of axillary surgery in patients with I-II carcinoma of the breast treated with primary radiotherapy. *Int J Radiat Oncol Biol Phys* 12:1575, 1986.

Stewart FW, and Treves N. Lymphangiosarcoma in post-mastectomy lymphedema: A report of six cases in elephantiasis chirurgica. *Cancer* 1:64, 1948.

Zucali R, et al. Contralateral breast cancer after limited surgery plus radiotherapy of early mammary tumors. *Eur J Surg Oncol* 13:413, 1989.

Radiation Therapy in the Augmented Breast

Halpern J, et al. Irradiation of prosthetically augmented breasts: A retrospective study on toxicity and cosmetic results. *Int J Radiat Oncol Biol Phys* 18:189, 1990.

Ryu J, et al. Radiation therapy after breast augmentation or reconstruction in early or recurrent breast cancer. *Cancer* 66:844, 1990.

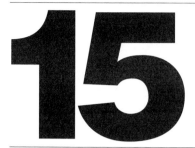

Adjuvant Therapy for Breast Cancer

Lois F. O'Grady

The lifetime risk of breast cancer for a woman living in North America is 1 in 9, up from the risk of 1 in 13 that existed only 10 years ago. The reasons for this increase are still speculative but include more effective and earlier diagnosis, an older population, and others unyet defined but which may include the prolonged menstrual life of twentieth-century women. This increased incidence has not escaped the attention of women, women's groups, and the lay (as well as medical) press—all of whom have been pushing for improved treatment strategies.

The acceptance of conservative approaches (i.e., lumpectomy and radiation therapy) to the primary lesion has been a major improvement in breast cancer therapy. A second improvement has been the development of treatment plans, such as chemotherapy and/or hormonal therapy, used as adjuncts to primary therapy in an attempt to improve the survival of patients.

The position of the U.S. National Cancer Institute is that all patients with breast cancer should receive adjuvant therapy. But many oncologists question the "all." These conflicting views, unfortunately, lead to confusion for the patient because she may hear one view from the surgeon, another from the radiation oncologist, and a third from the medical oncologist.

It is necessary to review some basic information about breast cancer—the therapeutic options available, the effectiveness of these therapies, and the negative impact of these therapies—before making some rational recommendations for consideration.

Background and Basics

Stages and Survival

Breast cancer can present with a barely detectable lesion, a huge fungating mass on the chest with widespread metastases, or anything in between. To help define groups for the purpose of comparison, invasive breast cancers are divided into stages I through IV. *Stage I* cancers are those that are less than 2 cm in diameter, are freely moveable in the breast, are not fixed to the skin or chest wall, and have not spread to the regional lymph nodes. *Stage II* cancers are larger tumors (up to 5 cm) that are confined to the breast, or tumors of any size up to 5 cm that have spread to the regional nodes. *Stage III* cancers are much larger and are sometimes inflammatory. Stage III cancers, because of their poor prognosis, are sometimes treated with aggressive multimodality therapy that is not customarily considered to be adjuvant therapy. Some of the smaller stage III cancers are treated with adjuvant therapy and for purposes of discussion can be considered with the stage II tumors. *Stage IV* cancers are metastatic at diagnosis. The therapy of metastatic cancer will not be addressed in this book.

Survival from cancer depends on the stage at diagnosis. A patient with stage I cancer has an 80% chance of being alive, free of disease, 5 years after diagnosis, her sister with stage II cancer has only a 60% chance, and someone in stage III has only a 40% chance. The figures for all will drop another 5% to 10% in 10 years.

This information provides us with some basic tumor biology: (1) breast cancer can spread beyond the local area even when the regional lymph nodes are not involved (indeed, we now consider the regional nodes to be just a marker of metastatic disease rather than a reflection of local growth), and (2) the distant spread can remain quiescent for long periods of time, suggesting it is a slow-growing tumor.

Note the phrase "alive, free of disease." In oncology there is a crucial distinction between "alive, free of disease," which implies potential curability, and "alive" (the fact of recurrent disease being unspoken) and probably not curable. The goal is cure but if that cannot be achieved, the second goal, of delayed recurrence and a few extra years of life without cancer, has merit.

Adjuvant Therapy for Stage II Disease

Several years ago, physicians began to ask whether there was anything that could be done to improve survival. At that time most patients presented with stage II disease. Some fairly successful chemotherapy drugs had become available, and it was known that these drugs were most effective against small volumes of tumor, as likely exist in these stage II patients just after surgery, in whom no tumor can be detected, but in whom cancer is destined to recur. Studies were begun in many areas of the world to determine if short courses of chemotherapy, given after surgery and as an adjunct to it, could improve the survival chances of patients.

The answer was yes. It took many years, many studies, and many heroic volunteers, but we have learned that if chemotherapy is given as combinations of two or three drugs (more are not necessary), for 6 months (longer isn't necessary), that there is a 25% decrease in mortality.

Let us consider that figure of 25%. It sounds too good to be true, and a careful look at how the figure was derived shows that it is.

Overall, among women with stage II breast cancer, there is a 36% mortality in the first 5 years. For those receiving adjuvant chemotherapy the mortality drops to 27%. Where's the 25%? The difference between 36% and 27% is 9% and 9 is 25% of 36. Nine represents the absolute number of extra survivors per 100 women treated. For those 9 of every 100 women, it is the difference between life and death.

The 25% represents a percentage reduction; the 9, an absolute reduction per 100 at risk. This difference between percent reduction and absolute reduction is an important concept to know when interpreting oncology studies.

Among the 27% of women who received the chemotherapy, but whose tumors recurred anyway, the recurrence was delayed by 18 to 24 months. That has some significance, because the physical and emotional quality of life during those 18 to 24 months was significantly better than after the tumor recurred.

What about the 64% of women who took the chemotherapy, and, statistically speaking, didn't need it? That is part of the cost/risk side of the equation we must examine next, to see if the benefit for the few was worth the risk imposed on the entire population.

Cost/Risk Versus Benefit

Let us look at a hypothetical group of 100 patients with stage II breast cancer. Statistically, 64 will be alive, free of disease in 5 years (and over 50 of them are cured). Thirty-six of them are destined for recurrent disease but if treatment is imposed on the whole group, 9 more will be cured and 27 will live a better life for 2 years. We cannot tell which patient belongs in which group, although the more risk factors for recurrence a woman has (see below), the greater the chance she will develop recurrence. Before we can decide if the risk-benefit ratio favors use of the treatment, we need to assess the risk and the cost.

Another very important concept that evolved from these studies was that the percentage risk reduction was the same in both the high-risk and low-risk groups. To illustrate this, let us examine two groups: one with a 50% chance of recurrence and one with a 20% chance of recurrence. If 50% of a group of 100 were to experience a recurrence, chemotherapy would decrease that number by 25% (50 × 0.25 = 12.5 individuals) or increase the number cured by 12.5 to 62.5%. But look at the low-risk group who had a 20% chance of recurrence and took the same chemotherapy. The risk decreased by 25% (20 × 0.25 = 5 individuals), and survival increased from 80% to 85%. *Although the risk of recurrence was different, and the chance of benefit was different, the cost of the chemotherapy for each individual in the population was fixed.*

What is this cost? It depends on whether the adjuvant therapy is hormonal or chemotherapeutic. Let us look at chemotherapy first.

Adjuvant chemotherapy for breast cancer is *relatively* easy in that the drugs used are among the least noxious of chemotherapeutic agents. There are, however, possible side effects including nausea, fatigue, hair loss, weight gain, and amenorrhea that may be permanent. With the newer drugs available to control symptoms, nausea should not be a major problem. Indeed, a year later, patients recall the fatigue as the most bothersome symptom. One must consider the costs of medical care and drugs, but also the hidden costs of days lost from work, babysitters, and transportation. About 1 in 20 patients will have serious side effects, for example, sepsis from pancytopenia. A few will even die (0.2%). In addition, all of the long-term sequelae may not be known. We do know that with the commonly used drugs (cyclophosphamide, methotrexate, and 5-fluorouracil) there is no increased incidence of secondary leukemias. There may be some late cardiac effects from Adriamycin, if that is used.

All these issues must be weighed against the chance for cure and delayed recurrence. If the risk of recurrence is 35%, and the risk of taking therapy is only 5%, the odds are in the patients favor. If, however, the risk of recurrence is 10%, Is it worth it?

Tables 15-1, 15-2, and 15-3 provide some figures that can help guide the decision whether adjuvant therapy is worth it. They show figures for both hormonal therapy (tamoxifen, which is discussed below) and chemotherapy. The risks of morbidity are shown as the percentage of patients who will experience symptoms severe enough to make them consider stopping the therapy; the mortality figures represent death during therapy. In Tables 15-2 and 15-3 the benefits are shown as two figures. The first figure (%) represents the percentage improvement in survival (reduction in mortality) as published in most of the literature. The number in parentheses represents the absolute number of extra survivors per 100 at risk, assuming that risk is 30% mortality in the population being studied. For example, in Table 15-2, under chemotherapy for women under 50 years, there is a 36% improvement in survival. If 30 women of every 100 are at risk of death, the absolute number of extra survivors is 11 (36% of 30). Note that Table 15-2 shows data relating to overall survival whereas Table 15-3, with the lower figures, shows survival free of disease and, thus, the possible cures achieved by the therapy.

In weighing factors for and against adjuvant therapy, the psychological set of the patient must be considered. Some patients are so fearful of chemotherapy that it would be counterproductive to insist on it; others are so fearful of the cancer that they want every possible thing done to improve their chances.

Although there are benefits to adjuvant chemotherapy, the costs are relatively high, and thus alternatives have been sought.

Alternatives to Chemotherapy

OOPHORECTOMY. It has been known since the 1940s that oophorectomy performed after breast cancer surgery delays recurrence but it was not thought to increase the cure rate. It was, in a way, a form

Table 15-1. Risks of adjuvant therapy

	Tamoxifen (%)	Chemotherapy (%)
Morbidity[a]	0	20
Mortality[b]	0.04	0.2

[a]Percentage of patients who experience side effects severe enough to make them consider stopping the therapy.
[b]Percentage of patients who die during therapy.

Table 15-2. Benefits of adjuvant therapy: improved 10-year survival*

	Tamoxifen	Chemotherapy
Age < 50	12% (4)	36% (11)
Age > 50	29% (9)	27% (8)
All ages	25% (7)	28% (8)

*The first figure represents the percentage improvement in survival (reduction in mortality). Figures in parentheses are absolute numbers of patients improved, assuming a 30% risk in the population studied.
Source: Data from the Early Breast Cancer Trialists' Collaborative Group (see three reports listed in Suggested Reading).

Table 15-3. Benefits of adjuvant therapy: improved 10-year disease-free survival*

	Tamoxifen	Chemotherapy
Age < 50	6% (2)	25% (7)
Age > 50	20% (6)	15% (4)
All ages	16% (5)	17% (5)

*The first figure represents the percentage improvement in survival (reduction in mortality). Figures in parentheses are absolute numbers of patients improved, assuming a 30% risk in the population studied.
Source: Data from the Early Breast Cancer Trialists' Collaborative Group (see three reports listed in Suggested Reading).

of adjuvant therapy. A recent review of oophorectomy by the Early Breast Cancer Trialists suggests that it is of more benefit than once thought, and it appears to truly cure some. In premenopausal women with node-negative disease, there is a 9.4% decrease in recurrence, and the decrease is 10.5% for patients with node-positive disease. The figures for decrease in mortality are 6.8% and 13%, respectively.

This new information has sparked great interest because the benefit appears great while the side effects of chemotherapy are not there. In the near future, we will see new trials combining oophorectomy with chemotherapy in an attempt to increase the beneficial results even more. At the present time, the oncology community is digesting this information and deciding whether to use oophorectomy more often. It would appear that oophorectomy is of more benefit in premenopausal women than tamoxifen.

TAMOXIFEN. As newer hormonal agents became available, they were tried as adjuvant therapies, primarily in women whose tumors contained receptors for estrogen and progesterone. The most widely used has been tamoxifen, an antiestrogen drug. It is given in a dosage of 10 mg twice a day for 5 years. It must be stressed that the favorable effects of tamoxifen adjuvant therapy are primarily for these hormone-receptor positive patients; in hormone-receptor negative patients the results, while still providing a measurable benefit, are less. Interestingly, it was thought that these antiestrogens would produce a "medical oophorectomy." In one sense they do, in that they block estrogenic effects on many tissues. In the presence of functioning ovaries, serum estrogen actually increases. This may be one reason that the drug is more effective in postmenopausal rather than premenopausal disease. It is not quite as effective as chemotherapy in the premenopausal patient but it does work. The number of cures are fewer, but the delay in recurrence is greater—3 to 4 years rather than 1½ years.

It is in the cost/risk versus benefit analysis that this therapy is attractive because its side effects are less severe than those of chemotherapy. Some side effects of tamoxifen include hot flashes in most women, vaginal dryness in 5% to 6%, vaginal discharge in 5% to 6%, and may carry a slight increased incidence of thromboembolic disease (*cf.* the early birth control pills), with a 0.04% risk of death. Tamoxifen increases the chances of developing endometrial cancer. A 1994 update of an NSABP trial of tamoxifen to treat breast cancer suggests an annual risk of 2 per 1000 women, or about 1% at 5 years. This level of risk is approximately 3 times greater than that for the general population and is about the same as for women taking estrogen for menopausal symptoms. This risk must be weighed carefully in the risk-benefit analysis. For the woman with breast cancer, the survival advantage with tamoxifen far outweighs the risk of a second cancer. For the woman taking tamoxifen for a few months (e.g., for fibrocystic disease) it is not a concern. Yearly pelvic examination should be routine. Routine endometrial biopsies are not recommended. However, transvaginal ultrasonographic examination of the uterus could be considered as a screening procedure for women on long-term tamoxifen therapy, beginning at the third year of therapy and every 2 to 3 years thereafter. If the endometrial lining is 4 mm or less in thickness, the presence of endometrial cancer is very unlikely. Abnormal bleeding or abnormal findings on physical or ultrasonographic examination should be evaluated with curettage or biopsy.

On the other hand, the benefits of tamoxifen are significant. Early concerns about osteoporosis have proved groundless. Indeed, the drug is actually a mixed agonist-antagonist drug, and its weak estrogen activity has maintained its users bone strength over many years of study. Similarly, concerns about estrogen withdrawal leading to increased heart disease also have proved false; the drug actually maintains a favorable lipid profile, and the incidence of ischemic cardiac events in treated patients has been half that of control-group patients. But the best news of all is that tamoxifen decreases the incidence of second breast cancers by 50%. Patients with one breast cancer have a 20% chance of developing a second cancer in the opposite breast (1% per year to a maximum of 20%), but in treated patients the change has been so significant that studies are under way in North America and Europe to evaluate the prophylactic use of the drug in women at high risk for breast cancer.

Will we now go back to oophorectomy instead of tamoxifen in premenopausal women? No. We'll probably use both—oophorectomy for more complete estrogen withdrawal and greater antitumor effect, and tamoxifen for its estrogeniclike beneficial effects on cardiovascular disease and bone density. It will take many years of study and many clinical trials to sort out the question of whether oophorectomy will replace chemotherapy or be used in combination with it.

Combination Chemotherapy and Hormonal Therapy

Although some studies are still under way, it appears that one can successfully use adjuvant chemotherapy immediately after primary therapy to achieve a higher percentage of cured patients, and then follow with prolonged administration of tamoxifen to achieve the longer-lasting recurrence delay and the added ancillary benefits of the drug. Using chemo- and hormonal therapy concurrently may increase toxicity (e.g., thromboembolic disease) without added benefit, thus, they should be used sequentially.

Combination Radiotherapy and Chemo-Hormonal Therapy

Radiation therapy is required as part of the conservative approach to management of primary breast cancer and may also be given following mastectomy if there is a high risk of local recurrence. Patients receiving radiotherapy often require adjuvant chemotherapy or hormonal therapy. There is no fixed schedule for delivery of the therapies, but it is difficult for most patients to receive chemotherapy and radiation therapy at the same time. In addition, there is evidence that some chemotherapy drugs (and perhaps also tamoxifen), given at the same time as the radiation, increase the risk of fibrosis.

Radiation therapy and chemotherapy are not usually given at the same time but there is no strong evidence to dictate the sequence. The decision is reached in consultation between the radiation and medical oncologists. Some give half of the chemotherapy first, then the radiation, and then the remainder of the chemotherapy— referred to as the "sandwich" technique. Other sequences have their proponents.

Adjuvant Therapy in Stage I Disease

Once it was established that chemotherapy and/or hormonal therapy was effective adjuvant treatment for stage II disease, it was not long before studies were begun to evaluate the same treatments for stage I disease. It would appear that chemotherapy or hormonal therapy provide the same percentage improvement for stage I patients, but because the numbers at risk are less, so are the improvements.

For example, in stage I disease there is 20% recurrence at 5 years. Chemotherapy will decrease that by the same 25% that we learned about in stage II disease, but instead of 20 patients in 100 developing recurrence, only 15 will. This represents a cure of 5 out of 100. However, the same 100 patients need to be treated to save the 5 and to prolong the disease-free survival of those 15 still destined to get recurrence. Therefore, the risk or cost to the population is that much higher: 80 are treated to no avail.

This increases the ethical and moral dilemma: Should treatments be offered to all patients? Should chemotherapy be reserved for the higher risk patients? Do we have the right to "harm" 80 in order to help 20? To help resolve this dilemma, a search was begun for those factors that might predict risk for recurrence.

Predictors of Recurrence

With the caveat that nothing is ever 100% true in medicine, there are several factors that can affect prognosis, as seen in Table 15-4.

1. *Invasiveness.* With the exception of large lesions (i.e., > 5 cm) that may harbor hidden areas of invasion, carcinomas in situ do not metastasize, and there is no need for adjuvant therapy.
2. *Size.* Tumors less than 1 cm in size rarely metastasize. In this group, the cost of adjuvant chemotherapy outweighs the benefit.
3. *Nodal status.* In patients with stage II disease, the more lymph nodes involved, the worse the prognosis.
4. *Hormone receptors.* Breast cancers vary tremendously in the number and avidity of cell membrane receptors for hormones (to use the common term *estrogen receptors* can be misleading because there are receptors for multiple hormones). The higher the level of receptors, the better behaved the tumor seems to be, that is, it recurs less often and if it does recur it does so much later. Patients with very low or negative hormone receptors carry

Table 15-4. Risk factors for recurrence

Factor	Lower risk	Higher risk
Size of tumor	Small	Large
Number of nodes	0–2	> 3
Hormone receptors	High	Low
Ploidy	Diploid	Aneuploid
S-phase	< 6	> 10

a worse prognosis. Hormone receptors were considered the primary risk determinant after tumor size and nodal status, but growth characteristics are now considered a more important prognostic factor.

5. *Growth characteristics.* Modern biomedical techniques allow us to quantify characteristics of tumors that were once referred to as well differentiated or poorly differentiated. We now assess the following characteristics on a routine basis:

    Ploidy. If the chromosome number of the tumor cells is normal (i.e., diploid), the tumors tend to be less aggressive. Chromosome numbers higher or lower than normal are aneuploid and carry a worse prognosis.

    S-phase. It is possible to determine what percent of the cells in a tumor are actively synthesizing DNA (i.e., in the S-phase). The more cells dividing, the higher the S-phase and the worse the prognosis. S-phase is turning out to be a powerful prognostic factor.

6. *Tumor markers.* A variety of enzymes and other proteins, such as cathepsins, and markers of oncogene expression, such as the Her-2-Neu oncogene, are being identified on cancers. At the present time there is no consensus on their predictive value and thus they should not be used routinely. In the near future, they may become more valuable tools.

A patient with a 0.5-cm stage I tumor, rich in hormone receptors, which is diploid and has a low S-phase, carries a much different prognosis than a patient with a 2-cm stage II tumor with negative hormone receptors, aneuploidy, and a high S-phase. The first needs no adjuvant therapy, the latter requires it. Those in the middle represent the challenge but the figures outlined in Tables 15-1 to 15-3 help guide decisions. Is the risk outlined in Table 15-1 worth the benefits noted in Tables 15-2 and 15-3?

Treatment Recommendations

Figures 15-1 and 15-2 outline the therapeutic approach to patients with stage I and stage II breast cancer, respectively. There are, however, some basic tenets about cancer therapy that first need review.

1. There is a great deal we do not know about cancer treatments. Patients should be encouraged to volunteer for national trials that offer state-of-the-art therapy and close monitoring of both the physician and the patient.

2. Patients should accept therapy only after significant consultation and after all of their questions have been answered. Informed consent is essential.

3. Patients have the right to participate in the selection of therapy when choices are available and the patient wishes to do so.

4. An absolute contraindication to chemotherapy is an uncoopera-

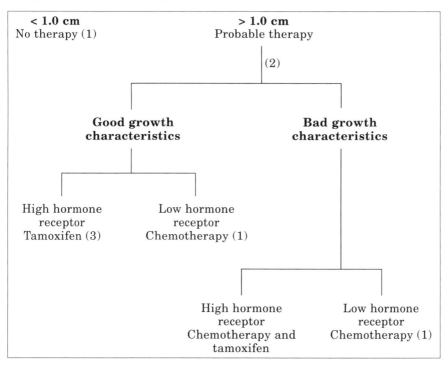

Fig. 15-1. Adjuvant therapy for stage I breast cancer. (1) = Consider tamoxifen prophylaxis (see text); (2) = If patient is premenopausal, consider oophorectomy (see text); (3) = In young patient, consider adding chemotherapy.

tive patient. The risk of early morbidity or mortality is too high to take the chance that a patient would treat a potentially lethal complication lightly.

5. Chemotherapy tends to have greater effect in patients under 50. Tamoxifen is more effective in patients over 50 with hormone-receptor positive tumors.

6. Hormonal therapy has fewer side effects and is less expensive than chemotherapy.

7. If a patient refuses chemotherapy, hormonal therapy is a viable alternative.

8. If a patient refuses all adjuvant therapy, she is worthy of respect, love, and continuing care.

Stage I Disease

For the patient with stage I disease (see Fig. 15-1) the major determinant of therapy is the size of the primary tumor. Tumors under 1 cm in size metastasize so rarely that the risk of any adjuvant therapy is higher than the risk of recurrence. Larger tumors have finite risks of recurrence; thus, adjuvant therapy is recommended. The type of adjuvant therapy depends on the character of the tumor. A tumor with unfavorable growth characteristics should be treated with mul-

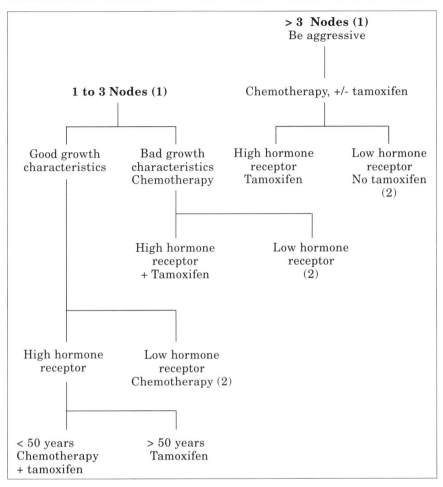

Fig. 15-2. Adjuvant therapy for stage II breast cancer. (1) = If patient is premenopausal, consider oophorectomy (see text); (2) = Consider tamoxifen prophylaxis.

tidrug chemotherapy for 4 to 6 months; if the tumor carries high levels of hormone receptors, chemotherapy should be followed by tamoxifen for 5 years.

There are ongoing clinical trials to determine the effectiveness of tamoxifen in women with hormone receptor–negative tumors. Preliminary results suggest a positive effect (although less than in hormone receptor–positive tumors) and in the near future all breast cancer patients may be treated with the drug either as therapy for the tumor or as prophylaxis against a second primary tumor.

Patients with tumors carrying favorable growth characteristics and high hormone receptors only need to receive tamoxifen, but if their hormone receptor status is low, the current recommendation is to use 6 months of chemotherapy.

On occasion, patients refuse chemotherapy or overriding medical or psychiatric factors prohibit its use. In such cases, use of tamoxifen, regardless of the patient's tumor characteristics, is better than no therapy at all.

Stage II Disease

All patients with stage II breast cancer should be offered adjuvant therapy. Decisions must be made as to the type of therapy. The survival statistics decrease dramatically when more than three nodes are involved; thus, that can be a starting point in the decision tree (see Fig. 15-2). Patients with more than three involved nodes should be treated as aggressively as possible because the risks of recurrence far outweigh the risks of chemotherapy. The use of tamoxifen after chemotherapy depends on the hormonal status of the tumor and the physician's philosophy about prophylactic tamoxifen in hormone receptor–negative women.

Patients with only a few nodes involved can be grouped according to the tumor's growth characteristics. Unfavorable factors require aggressive therapy. If the tumor has favorable growth factors and a high hormone–receptor status, the patient could be treated with tamoxifen alone. In Britain, she would be. In the United States, current recommendations are to use chemotherapy in women under the age of 50 and probably in the 50- to 60-year-old age group as well, followed by tamoxifen. Antiestrogen alone would be used in the older group. Here again, patient preference can help in the decisions.

Summary

In summary, very small tumors (i.e., < 1 cm) need no adjuvant treatment. Stage I diploid tumors with low S-phase (favorable growth characteristics) may be treated with hormonal agents alone. Other patients diagnosed with stage I breast cancer may benefit from chemotherapy with or without tamoxifen.

All stage II patients should receive adjuvant therapy. Tamoxifen alone can be used for tumors with high receptor levels and good growth factors (see Table 15-4), especially in women over 50. All others should receive 6 months of multiagent chemotherapy, with or without tamoxifen to follow.

Suggested Reading

Predictors of Recurrence

Carter CL, Allen C, and Henson DE. Relation of tumor size, lymph node status, and survival in 24,740 breast cancer cases. *Cancer* 63: 181–187, 1989.

Clark GM, et al. Prediction of relapse or survival in patients with node-negative breast cancer by DNA flow cytometry. *N Engl J Med* 320:627–633, 1989.

Clark GM, et al. Prognostic significance of S-phase fraction in good risk, node negative breast cancer patients. *J Clin Oncol* 10:428–432, 1992.

McGuire WL, et al. How to use prognostic factors in axillary node-negative breast cancer patients. *J Natl Cancer Inst* 82:1006–1015, 1990.

Benefits of Therapy

Bonnadonna G, and Valagussa P. Systemic therapy in resectable breast cancer. *Hematol Oncol Clin North Am* 3:727–742, 1989.

Early Breast Cancer Trialists' Collaborative Group. Effects of adjuvant tamoxifen and cytotoxic therapy on mortality in early breast cancer. *N Engl J Med* 319:1681–1692, 1988.

Early Breast Cancer Trialists' Collaborative Group. *Worldwide Evidence 1985–1990.* Vol. 1 of Treatment of Early Breast Cancer. New York: Oxford University Press, 1990.

Early Breast Cancer Trialists' Collaborative Group. Systemic treatment of early breast cancer by hormonal, cytotoxic, or immune therapy: 133 randomized trials involving 31,000 recurrences and 24,000 deaths among 75,000 women. *Lancet* 339(8784):1–15, 71–85, 1992.

Rosner D, Lane WW. Should all patients with node-negative breast cancer receive adjuvant therapy? *Cancer* 68:1482–1494, 1991.

Tamoxifen

Bagdale JD, et al. Effects of tamoxifen treatment on plasma lipids and lipoprotein composition. *J Clin Endocrinol Metab* 70:1132–1135, 1990.

Fornander T, et al. Long-term adjuvant tamoxifen in early breast cancer: Effect on bone mineral density in post menopausal women. *J Clin Oncol* 8:1019–1024, 1991.

Love RR, et al. Effects of tamoxifen on bone mineral density in post-menopausal women with breast cancer. *N Engl J Med* 326:852–856, 1992.

Love RR, et al. Effects of tamoxifen therapy on lipid and lipoprotein levels in post-menopausal patients with node-negative breast cancer. *J Natl Cancer Inst* 82:1327–1332, 1990.

McDonald CC, and Stewart HJ. Fatal myocardial infarction in the Scottish adjuvant tamoxifen trial. *Br Med J* 303:435–437, 1991.

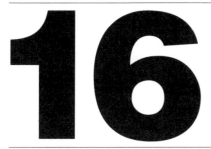

16

Breast Cancer in Pregnancy

Mary B. Rippon

During pregnancy the breast undergoes more dramatic changes than those experienced monthly during the menstrual cycle. An increase in breast size and tenderness is often noted early in the first trimester and may be a woman's first indication of pregnancy. As the pregnancy progresses, the breasts become firmer and more nodular in preparation for lactation. The physiologic changes that occur in the breast during pregnancy and lactation are described in Chap. 1.

Breast Examination During Pregnancy

Examination of the breast during pregnancy becomes more difficult for both the patient and the health practitioner because of the natural changes that are occurring in the breast. The importance of a good baseline breast examination as well as regular follow-up examinations cannot be stressed enough. A mass present prior to the pregnancy can be masked easily by the subsequent physiologic changes that occur during pregnancy. The breast should be examined both in the sitting and supine positions, just as in the nongravid patient (see Chap. 7). Extension of the arm above the head in the supine position will flatten the tissue against the chest wall, making the breast easier to examine. The breasts will naturally demonstrate increased nodularity on examination, but a single, unilateral, dominant mass requires attention.

The patient should continue monthly breast self-examination throughout pregnancy. Breast examination by the health practitioner should be performed regularly as well; this can be done in conjunction with the monthly obstetric visit. The primary problem with breast cancer in pregnancy is delay in diagnosis, resulting in women being diagnosed with breast cancer during pregnancy at a later (i.e., more advanced) stage.

The Palpable Mass During Pregnancy

For most women pregnancy is a time filled with joy, anticipation, and a degree of natural anxiety. When a mass is found by either the patient or her physician a sudden shadow of fear may be cast on this special time and the woman's anxiety exponentially increased. On the other hand, the patient or practitioner may dismiss the mass completely, considering it normal and to be expected during pregnancy. Although the vast majority of "lumps" encountered during pregnancy are benign and transient, it is imperative that the possibility of a malignancy be considered.

Benign masses that may occur during pregnancy and lactation include cysts, fibroadenomas, lactating adenomas, galactoceles, and breast infarcts. Preexisting fibroadenomas may increase in size and become tender due to the hormonal stimulation of pregnancy.

Evaluation of the Palpable Mass

Evaluation of a mass found in a pregnant woman is similar in many ways to that in the nongravid patient (see Figs. 7-1 and 7-4). Concern for the unborn fetus, of course, should always be demonstrated. The size, texture, and mobility of the mass should be described as should any change from previous exams. Any changes in the nipple, such as retraction or bloody discharge, should also be noted.

Ultrasound

After the physical examination, a breast ultrasound may be helpful in the evaluation. A *galactocele,* or milk-filled cyst, may appear as a thick-walled mass of fluids of different densities due to the separation of fat and milk. This appearance, when it occurs, is distinctive and can be differentiated from homogeneous solid masses such as cancers and fibroadenomas. There is no radiation exposure during ultrasound, and it is a procedure the patient may be familiar with from the fetal ultrasounds performed during pregnancy. Fine needle aspiration (FNA) or core needle biopsy also can be performed, with ultrasound guidance, to demonstrate those lesions that are difficult to palpate.

Mammography

A mammogram of the breast with the palpable mass can be done safely in pregnancy if the fetus is adequately shielded. Generally, the mammogram can provide better definition of the palpable abnormality and evaluates the remainder of ipsilateral and contralateral breast for the presence of multifocal disease. Although mammography is the gold standard for screening and diagnosis of breast disease, in pregnancy its sensitivity may be decreased due to the increased breast density. Mammography should be done before surgical biopsy because the procedure will cause postoperative changes that potentially distort the architecture of the breast parenchyma making the mammogram more difficult to interpret.

Fine Needle Aspiration

Fine needle aspiration can be used to distinguish a cystic mass from a solid one and can provide a cytologic diagnosis of the solid mass.

Fine needle aspirates from the pregnant or lactating breast need to be interpreted by an experienced cytopathologist because the hormonally induced hyperplasia that occurs with pregnancy and lactation can demonstrate atypical cytologic features similar to carcinoma. The pathologist should be made aware of the patient's clinical history so that these cellular changes can be placed in the appropriate context.

If aspiration reveals either clear cystic fluid or the milklike fluid of a galactocele, and the mass resolves with aspiration, no other intervention is required. If the mass does not resolve with aspiration, excisional biopsy should be considered. A solid mass with benign cytology (e.g., fibroadenoma) that is not excised requires close scrutiny. The patient should be reexamined in 3 to 4 weeks, with examinations repeated monthly throughout the pregnancy. If the mass increases in size, excisional biopsy should be performed despite a benign cytologic diagnosis. Fine needle aspiration results that are suspicious, atypical, insufficient, or nondiagnostic require further evaluation with excisional biopsy.

Excisional Biopsy

An excisional biopsy can be performed safely at any time during pregnancy as an outpatient procedure using local anesthesia. If the patient is close to the end of her first trimester, when organogenesis occurs and the highest risk of miscarriage exists even without intervention, the surgeon may elect to defer the biopsy until the beginning of the second trimester. This precaution is unnecessary—the diagnosis of a suspicious mass should not be delayed.

Concern about the development of *milk fistulas* after breast biopsy during lactation has led some surgeons to suppress lactation pharmacologically prior to the procedure. Milk fistula is rarely a clinical problem, especially if the lesion is located peripherally in the breast and suppression is not necessary in most cases.

Breast Cancer in Pregnancy

Carcinoma of the breast is the most common malignancy to occur during pregnancy. The incidence of breast cancer during pregnancy has been reported as being between 1 in 3000 and 1 in 10,000 pregnancies. The incidence of breast cancer increases with age; given that more women are choosing to delay childbearing, we may see the incidence of breast cancer during pregnancy increase as well.

A breast cancer diagnosed during pregnancy is terrifying and can change the whole focus of the pregnancy. Breast cancer, however, can be treated adequately during pregnancy; termination of the pregnancy is *not* required. Should the patient wish to terminate the pregnancy, the treatment options would of course be the same as for the nongravid patient (see Chap. 14). Termination of the pregnancy does *not* improve patient survival.

Once a pregnant woman has been diagnosed with breast cancer, at least a limited staging work-up, including a mammogram and blood tests, should be done. The serologic tests should include a complete blood count (CBC) and chemistry panel with liver function tests. The liver function tests provide a basic screen for liver metastases and bone metastases with the inclusion of the alkaline phosphatase levels, although the pregnancy itself may cause some elevation in the alkaline phosphatase. Some oncologists also order a cancer antigen 15-3 (CA 15-3), which is a new marker for breast cancer that may be used in the future in a fashion similar to carcinoembryonic antigen (CEA). CA 15-3 measurement, however, is not very sensitive in early breast cancer and its use is not yet supported by the Food and Drug Administration (FDA).

A mammogram of both breasts is needed before any definitive surgery is performed to rule out multifocal or contralateral disease. Once again, the fetus needs to be adequately shielded. A chest x-ray that is ordinarily performed in the routine staging of breast cancer may be excluded in the pregnant woman to decrease any unnecessary exposure, especially if the patient appears to have an early-stage breast cancer.

For those patients presenting with clinically advanced disease (e.g., mass > 5 cm, axillary adenopathy, skin involvement) some of the tests considered routine for metastatic screening in the nongravid situation (see Table 14-2) may be omitted to avoid undue radiation exposure. An ultrasound of the liver can be done to rule out metastases but a bone scan or abdominal CT should be deferred unless the results would affect the patient's decision regarding pregnancy termination and treatment options.

The treatment of a woman diagnosed with breast cancer during pregnancy should *not* be delayed unless she is within 2 to 3 weeks of her scheduled delivery date.

Treatment Options

In considering treatment options for the pregnant woman with breast cancer, two factors must be kept in mind. First, radiation therapy is not offered because of the potential scatter to the fetus, despite shielding, when 5400 cGy (rads) are being given to the breast. Second, chemotherapy choices are limited. All chemotherapy drugs should be avoided in the first half of pregnancy. However, once organogenesis is complete and the pregnancy is well established, certain chemotherapeutic agents can be administered safely. Hormonal therapy (e.g., tamoxifen) should be avoided during the pregnancy due to the potential teratogenic effects on the fetus.

First and Second Trimesters

Modified radical mastectomy is the primary treatment for patients in their first or second trimester. Breast conservation, which includes lumpectomy, axillary node dissection, and radiation therapy, is not advocated because of the risk from radiation to the fetus. In breast-conserving therapy without breast irradiation, the risk of recurrence in the breast is as high as 40%. The risk of delaying the radiation for many months until after delivery is uncertain, but an increased risk of recurrence would be expected when compared to the standard of starting the radiation therapy 4 to 6 weeks after surgery. The purpose of radiation therapy after breast-conserving surgery is to treat the remainder of the breast for potential areas of preinvasive or multifocal disease; those potential areas of subclinical premalignant disease would be under continued hormonal stimulation throughout the duration of the pregnancy. It is for these reasons that modified radical mastectomy is the standard treatment for breast cancer diagnosed during the first or second trimester of pregnancy provided that the patient wishes to maintain the pregnancy. Consideration of reconstruction is best delayed until the conclusion of pregnancy and lactation, when the breasts have decreased to a normal and stable size. The appropriate symmetry between the reconstructed breast and the native breast can then be attained.

Third Trimester

The woman who is diagnosed with breast cancer in the third trimester has several treatment options. If she is very close to term, surgery may be delayed for 1 to 2 weeks until after delivery or labor can be induced as soon as the fetus is mature. The decision to induce labor is clearly made in conjunction with the patient's obstetrician and may be as early as 2 to 4 weeks before the projected delivery date.

If breast cancer is diagnosed at the beginning of the third trimester, definitive surgery should be done at that time. This surgery may be either a modified radical mastectomy *or* a lumpectomy and axillary node dissection with radiation therapy delayed until after delivery. Chemotherapy also may be delayed until after delivery. Because chemotherapeutic drugs may be secreted in breast milk, the patient should not breastfeed in conjunction with chemotherapy.

In women who have poor prognostic signs, such as large tumors, multiple positive nodes, or inflammatory carcinoma, early induction of labor or immediate initiation of chemotherapy if it is too early for induction of labor should be considered. There should be no risk to the fetus from appropriate chemotherapy during this time. Reconstruction should not be done until the breasts have resumed their normal size.

Surgical Considerations

When surgery is performed in the second half of pregnancy, there are several helpful techniques to keep in mind:

1. Pregnant women have delayed gastric emptying; therefore, when general anesthesia is used, a *rapid sequence induction* should be considered. This technique, which is used frequently in anesthesia, anticipates the presence of a full stomach.

2. In the later stages of pregnancy, a pillow should be placed under the patient's right side to tilt her toward the left; this shifts the weight of the enlarged uterus off the vena cava and thus improves venous return.

3. *Fetal monitoring* keeps a watchful eye on the baby during the procedure.

Termination of an early pregnancy for breast cancer is not necessary, but is an option that some women may want to consider. Termination of the pregnancy does not improve the prognosis of the breast cancer, but it does change the therapeutic options. If a woman presents with an aggressive or advanced breast cancer (e.g., multiple nodes, large mass, metastatic disease), the pregnancy may dissuade or delay aggressive multimodality treatment with chemo- and radiation therapy that might otherwise be indicated based on the extent of disease.

Fetal Risk

The potential risks to the fetus from the treatments offered have been noted above. In general, hormonal therapy and radiation therapy are not recommended while the fetus is still in utero. Surgery, however, can be performed at any time during pregnancy. For women diagnosed in the latter part of the first trimester, it may be preferable to hold off the definitive surgery under a general anesthetic until the second trimester *if* it does not result in undue delay in treatment. This is merely an added precaution to avoid the period of organogenesis. The biopsy, however, can be done under local anesthesia and should not be deferred. If indicated, selected chemotherapeutic agents may be given safely in the third trimester. There is no risk of the breast cancer being transmitted to the fetus through the placenta.

Remember, *the greatest risk to the baby is a delay in diagnosis of the mother,* leading to a more advanced stage of cancer and a worse prognosis.

Prognosis

There are conflicting reports in the literature as to whether the prognosis of breast cancer during pregnancy is worse or the same as in the nongravid woman. Because the numbers are small, studies tend to be retrospective and to include patients diagnosed during pregnancy as well as in the year following pregnancy. Often the series have been accumulated over a long period of time during which both treatment modalities and the aggressivenes of the disease may have changed.

Several authors conclude that when matched for age and stage, pregnant women with breast cancer have the same prognosis as nongravid women. Conversely, an article by Guinee, et al. reports a significantly less favorable prognosis for the pregnant patient with breast cancer in the 20- to 29-year-old age group. This age group represents a very small subset of breast cancer patients.

Much remains to be learned about breast cancer in pregnancy. We know that it usually takes several years for a breast cancer to grow to the point that it is clinically detectable. It is unknown whether the hormonal changes of pregnancy stimulate cancer growth or have the ability to cause an area of atypia or carcinoma in situ to develop into an invasive lesion. Further studies to address the question of tumor biology and to determine prognosis are needed. Ideally a prospective study should be done, but this may be difficult with limited numbers of these patients at any one institution.

The greatest rectifiable problem with breast cancer in pregnancy is delay in diagnosis. All of the reported series consistently show patients diagnosed during pregnancy to be at a more advanced stage than comparable nongravid patients. The incidence of nodal positivity in pregnant women with breast cancer is nearly double that in the nongravid patient (70–80% versus 40%). Node-positive breast cancer does carry a worse prognosis than node-negative breast cancer with an increased recurrence rate and decreased overall survival.

In conclusion, early detection and avoidance of undue delays in treatment of breast cancer in pregnant women are the only known means to improve prognosis.

Suggested Reading

Barnavon Y, and Wallack MK. Collective reviews: Management of the pregnant patient with carcinoma of the breast. *Surg Gynecol Obstet* 171:347, 1990.

Clark RM, and Chua T. Breast cancer and pregnancy: The ultimate challenge. *Clin Oncol* 1:11, 1989.

Guinee VF, et al. Effect of pregnancy on prognosis for young women with breast cancer. *Lancet* 343:1587, 1994.

Hoover HC. Breast cancer during pregnancy and lactation. *Surg Clin North Am* 70:1151, 1990.

Petrek JA. Pregnancy-associated breast cancer. *Sem Surg Oncol* 7:306d, 1991.

Petrek JA, Dukoff R, and Rogatko A. Prognosis of pregnancy-associated breast cancer. *Cancer* 67:866, 1991.

Titcomb CL. Breast cancer and pregnancy. *Hawaii Med J* 49:18, 1990.

Van der Vange N, and van Dongen JA. Breast cancer and pregnancy. *Eur J Surg Oncol* 17:1, 1991.

Zemlickis D, et al. Maternal and fetal outcome after breast cancer in pregnancy. *Am J Obstet Gynecol* 166:781–787, 1992.

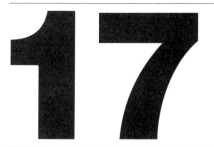

Expectations of Therapy

Lois F. O'Grady
and Janice K. Ryu

Any procedure or treatment affecting the breast causes patients great concern because most do not know what to expect from the planned investigation or treatment. This chapter addresses the anatomic, functional, and cosmetic results to be expected after investigative procedures and therapy to the breast.

Investigations and Biopsies

Fine Needle Aspiration

Fine needle aspiration (FNA) has become popular because it provides rapid diagnosis, is cost-effective, and lacks complications. There is minimal tenderness, an occasional bruise, and rare cases of infection. The patients return to normal functioning the same day. If the FNA is done to investigate a mass, the mass remains, unless cystic fluid is removed.

Core Needle Biopsy

With core needle biopsy (see Chap. 5), there is a greater chance of hematoma than with FNA, and the breast may be sore for a day or two. Infection is rare and there will be no scar. The patient should return to normal functioning the same day. The biopsied mass will remain.

Open Biopsy

Open biopsy is performed for a palpable mass or after a needle localization for a nonpalpable, mammographically detected abnormality. It is an outpatient surgery usually performed under local anesthesia with sedation. Although the breast may be sore for several days, the need for more than mild analgesia (acetaminophen with or without codeine) to relieve discomfort is rare. A hematoma may result, filling the underlying cavity with serous or serosanguineous fluid that may drain through the incision. With time, the breast tissue remolds itself to fill the cavity. There will be a scar but infection is uncommon. Patients can generally resume normal functioning the next day but strenuous exercise should be avoided for several days to allow wound healing. The breast may (or may not) have local induration for several weeks; if it does, the patient may need reassurance. Breast function and sensation will be normal.

Open biopsy may be incisional or excisional. If the surgeon is suspicious of malignancy, a wide rim of normal tissue may be taken from around the lesion. This is known as a lumpectomy and is discussed later in the chapter.

Biopsies are done to exclude malignancy; thus, these patients are under great stress. Results of pathology reports should be communicated quickly. If malignancy is found, the patient should be seen immediately for counseling.

If the pathology shows high-risk changes such as atypical hyperplasia or lobular carcinoma in situ, the patient will need a careful explanation of the significance of the findings (see Chaps. 12 and 13) and may need counseling if she overreacts to the diagnosis and lives in fear of cancer. She also deserves a detailed plan for follow-up.

Duct Excision

The major ductal structures of one or both breasts may need to be excised to treat repeat infections of the nipple-areolar complex from comedomastitis, to investigate a bloody discharge, or to remove a papilloma. Duct excision is outpatient surgery. The breast may be sore for several days and a hematoma may develop. The risk of infection is small. The incision (and resulting scar) usually can be made at the edge of the areola where it is cosmetically acceptable. Depending on the amount of tissue removed, a small structural defect (a "hole") under the nipple may occur, and some nipple sensation may be lost. Nursing still may be possible if only one or two ducts are excised. To treat comedomastitis, the entire ductal complex is removed, and nursing is not possible. Because comedomastitis is a disease of women in their forties, this does not generally pose a problem.

Therapeutic Procedures

Lumpectomy

Lumpectomy removes the lesion and an adequate margin, usually at least 1 cm, of normal tissue around the lesion. It is done as outpatient surgery. The degree of soreness, hematoma formation, and induration is directly related to the amount of tissue removed. To relieve soreness the patient will require analgesia; a preparation containing codeine, oxycodone (e.g., Percodan), or hydrocodone (e.g., Vicodin) will suffice. The major soreness eases in 2 to 3 days and should be gone in 10 days. A linear scar will remain. A small biopsy from a generous-sized breast may leave no defect because the cavity will fill with seroma fluid and the breast tissue will remold with time. A large biopsy in a small breast may leave some defect; the size of the defect is determined by the size of the lesion and the size of the breast. The aim of lumpectomy is to remove the lesion while preserving cosmesis; thus, if the surgeon anticipates removal of more than 25% of the breast, mastectomy with or without reconstruction will be recommended instead. In a few breast centers, teams of breast surgeons and plastic surgeons are developing techniques for partial mastectomy with immediate reconstruction, prior to radiation therapy, but this is not generally available.

If no subsequent treatment is given, the breast will be functional. However, if radiation therapy is given it will destroy breast parenchyma, so it will not be possible to nurse from the treated breast. Nursing should be possible from the untreated breast. Centrally located tumors may necessitate removal of the nipple-areolar complex, after which nursing is not possible.

Lymph Node Dissection

Lymph node dissection is now commonly done with lumpectomy and requires a separate incision in the axilla, rather than being a continuation of the lumpectomy incision. Structurally and cosmetically this is better because there is less deformity and less limitation of movement. Even so, the surgery may produce a significant anatomic defect that should not be evident unless the arm is raised.

Permanent paresthesia of the axilla and inner upper arm can result from lymph node dissection. There is some risk of residual lymphedema (less than 10%); this risk is now less than it was because the uppermost nodes (level 3) are no longer removed routinely. If radiation therapy is delivered to the axilla, the risk of edema increases. Standard radiotherapy for breast cancer, however, excludes the axilla unless extensive tumor is found.

Patients are discharged from the hospital, often the next day, with a drain (or drains) in place. Once the drain(s) is removed, 7 to 10 days later, the patient may begin to exercise. Indeed, she should be encouraged to exercise the arm to prevent any limitation of motion. Full range of motion should be achieved in 1 month. Some patients may benefit from the assistance of a physical therapist. The expectation is for full recovery of mobility and full resumption of normal activities (e.g., swimming, tennis, or golf).

Because the lymphatic drainage is disturbed, the arm is at increased risk of infection. Penetrating wounds, including phlebotomy, are to be avoided. Any skin infection should be treated promptly with antibiotics. The increased risk of infection is lifelong. Patients should take simple precautions such as wearing gloves while gardening.

Mastectomy

Most patients who have a mastectomy are able to leave the hospital after 2 to 3 days; some even leave on the first postoperative day. Drains are in place, and patients are instructed to keep a daily log of the drainage. When it is less than 30 cc per day, usually 7 to 10 days later, the drains are removed. The patients should begin an exercise program and can expect full range of motion of the arm and shoulder by 1 month. The patient may notice numbness near the scar once the wound heals and over the course of several months may notice some paresthesias over the chest wall as the local nerves regenerate.

While in the hospital, the patient should be referred to the American Cancer Society Reach to Recovery Program (see Chap. 21). Their hospital or home visit will provide the patient with her initial prosthesis as well as advice on local sources for prostheses. As soon as the chest wall is healed (2–4 weeks), the patient should begin to wear a well-fitted and weighted prosthesis as much for posture as for cosmesis.

Radiation Therapy

Radiation therapy is given to the intact breast of all patients after lumpectomy. After mastectomy, only selected patients will require radiation therapy depending on the number of nodes involved with tumor and the presence or absence of lymphatic and/or vascular invasion. In these patients the radiation may be delivered to the chest wall, ipsilateral supraclavicular fossa, axilla, or any combination of the three.

Skin Reaction

During the course of radiation therapy, which lasts 4 to 6 weeks, the patient can expect varying degrees of skin reaction—anything from slight erythema to moist desquamation. The severity depends on several factors.

1. Similar to sunburn, radiation dermatitis is most severe in patients with a light complexion; the patient's history of sunburn may predict to what degree their breast skin will react to radiation.
2. Patients with pendulous breasts with large skin folds in the axillary tail and inframammary fold may develop desquamation in those areas.
3. Treatment techniques can also affect the skin reaction. The use of modern megavoltage equipment, with its skin-sparing property, has greatly reduced the incidence of severe acute or chronic skin changes. However, the use of electrons, either for a boost or for chest wall irradiation, may deliver a high enough skin dose to cause dry or moist desquamation. Poor matching technique

between radiation fields can produce an overlap causing matchline desquamation and later fibrosis.

4. Certain substances (referred to as *bolus material*), when applied to the skin, can increase the skin dose of radiation, increasing effectiveness but at the same time causing a worse skin reaction.

The majority of patients will experience a mild to moderate degree of erythema and patchy dry desquamation by the time therapy is completed.

Radiation effects on the skin depend on the total accumulative dose given to the skin; therefore most patients do not develop problems nor do they require intervention until the fourth or fifth week of therapy. When erythema or dryness occurs, we recommend that the patient apply moisturizing creams or ointments. Pruritus and dry desquamation may be managed symptomatically with topical dusting of cornstarch or baby powder. Patients are instructed to wash off all powder, creams, and ointments before daily treatment to avoid a buildup that could function as bolus material. Redness subsides in several weeks following the completion of radiation therapy. Tanning, however, may not disappear for many months.

A small minority of patients develop moist desquamation, requiring a week to 10-day treatment break. This can be managed with a topical wound dressing (e.g., Sorbsan) that forms a hydrophilic gel and provides an environment that is both conducive to healing and soothing to the patient. Mild analgesia may be required (e.g., codeine, oxycodone).

Edema

The majority of patients undergoing breast irradiation notice edema of the treated breast. The breast may feel heavy or tense. Breast edema usually subsides within 3 months of radiation therapy, although edema may last significantly longer in some large breasts.

Severe or symptomatic arm edema is uncommon with modern surgical procedures, unless axillary irradiation is combined with extensive (levels 1, 2, and 3) axillary dissection. The treatment of arm edema starts with a light elastic sleeve and an exercise regimen. The swelling may decrease with weight loss in heavy patients. Those patients with severe edema should be referred to physical therapy for instruction in special exercises and in the use of a pneumocompression sleeve (see Appendix C). Strenuous exercises are to be avoided and injury and infections of the edematous arm prevented.

Other Complications

Chronic complications are rare if proper breast irradiation technique is used. When radiation ports are not matched precisely and reproducibly at each treatment session, matchline fibrosis between fields can produce a poor cosmetic result. Other rare late side effects include delayed radiation-induced chest wall muscle inflammation, which causes tenderness. This side effect is self-limited and resolves promptly with the use of nonsteroidal antiinflammatory drugs.

Radiation may also weaken ribs in the treated area and can cause rib fracture 1 to 2 years following radiation therapy. Radiation-induced rib fractures are often asymptomatic and can be treated conservatively. They may show on bone scans, however, and can be confused with metastases by the unwary.

Radiation may cause inflammation of the lung if too much lung is included in the tangential breast fields. Radiation pneumonitis occurs 6 weeks to 3 months following radiation therapy. Its severity depends on the volume of lung in the radiation ports. Patients may complain of shortness of breath, dry cough, and low grade fever. The chest x-ray will reveal consolidation in the periphery of the lung fields corresponding exactly to the radiation ports. This complication is rare (less than 2% of patients) and self-limiting. An occasional patient will require treatment with steroids, 20 to 30 mg of prednisone per day for a week or so, with rapid taper. The volume of lung irradiated is only a small fraction of the total lung capacity (well under 10%) and, in most patients, breast irradiation has no impact on lung function in the long run.

The breast does not lactate after whole breast irradiation for cancer. Child-bearing women undergoing breast-conserving therapy should be made aware of this fact. The contralateral breast, however, does lactate and the woman should be able to nurse from that side.

Other Risks

Most epidemiologic studies reveal no higher contralateral breast cancer risk in those who opted for breast-conserving therapy (which includes breast irradiation) compared to those treated with mastectomy. However, one recent study found that in women less than 45 years of age, there was a small but significant increase in the incidence of contralateral breast cancer in women treated with lumpectomy and radiation therapy compared to women treated with mastectomy. The same study found no increase in the contralateral breast cancer risk for those over 45 years of age. This is not surprising because we know that breast cancer risk is increased in women who, during their early years (i.e., breast development years), received low-dose radiation from repeated fluoroscopies.

There is no evidence that radiation therapy of the breast or chest wall induces any other type of tumor.

Adjuvant Chemotherapy

The drugs used for adjuvant therapy of breast cancer are potent, but not the most onerous chemotherapeutic agents for the patient to take. With judicious use of prochlorperazine (Compazine), lorazepam (Ativan), dexamethasone (Decadron, a centrally active antinauseant), and the new antiserotonin drugs like ondansetron (Zofran), nausea and vomiting are minimal. Many patients compare the nausea to the morning sickness of pregnancy. Some patients are sleepy for several hours after the chemotherapy from the antinauseants but otherwise are able to continue working, traveling, and even driving.

Hair loss begins about 3 weeks after the chemotherapy starts. It may be complete but almost always regenerates. The regrowth is usually in the same natural color but (surprisingly) often has more natural curl.

Fatigue is more of a problem than nausea; patients report functioning at about 75% of normal. Most patients find that they go to bed earlier, rest more, and are less active. Many women, however, continue their employment and their family responsibilities with no extra assistance. The amount of fatigue varies, of course, from patient to patient. Energy levels return to normal about 1 month after the chemotherapy is finished. Patients are encouraged to be as active as they wish and to maintain a regular exercise program, although it may need to be more limited than usual.

Weight gain (yes, gain) may be significant. Many patients gain over 10 pounds, probably the result of increased snacking to quiet an uneasy stomach and decreased activity.

Menstrual irregularities including amenorrhea are common because the drugs affect ovarian function. If the patient is under 35, menses may resume within 6 months of completion of therapy. The closer the patients are to the menopause, the more likely the amenorrhea is to be permanent. Remember, *amenorrhea does not necessarily mean infertility; thus, birth control measures are mandatory* because the drugs are potentially teratogenic.

Estrogen replacement may or may not be in the best interest of the patient (see Chap. 10). Regular weight-bearing exercise, along with 1500 mg of calcium daily, and perhaps a daily dose of 20 μg/day (400 IU) of vitamin D are prudent recommendations.

The fatigue, hair loss, and chronic low-grade malaise can lead to depression. Careful inquiry should be made to determine if the patient or family members are experiencing early signs of clinical depression (e.g., altered sleep, crying spells, mood alterations) so that counseling can be arranged. Most hospitals have social workers who can be helpful and most local American Cancer Society offices have lists of support groups. These support groups are very helpful and often offer exercise programs as well as advice on general health and beauty (see Appendix C).

Adjuvant Hormonal Therapy

Adjuvant hormonal therapy may be the only adjuvant therapy or it may follow a course of chemotherapy. Tamoxifen is the agent most commonly prescribed. It is actually a mixed agonist-antagonist drug, acting as an antiestrogen in some tissues and mimicking estrogen in others. It is extraordinarily well tolerated. Recent evidence documents its estrogenlike effect on bone density, its favorable lipid profiles, and its protection against ischemic heart disease. The most common complaint with tamoxifen use are hot flashes. These are worse in some and better tolerated by others. Antihistamines (e.g., diphenhydramine), atropinic drugs (e.g., Bellergal-S), and antihypertensives (e.g., clonidine) may be helpful, as detailed in Chap. 18. As occurs in normal menopause, the hot flashes abate with time in most women. Other side effects are reviewed in Chap. 15.

Pregnancy

In years gone by, the idea of pregnancy in a patient with a history of breast cancer was taboo because of the fear that growth of the breast induced by pregnancy would induce growth of the cancer already present or growth of an incipient cancer in the opposite breast. It was also thought that the advanced stage of breast cancers found in pregnancy resulted from the high hormone levels present in pregnancy.

In recent years, demographic changes and new knowledge have led to a rethinking of this issue. More women are postponing pregnancies until their late thirties, more breast cancers are being diagnosed in women in their thirties, and more breast cancers are small, giving patients an 80% to 90% chance of long-term survival. There is therefore a cohort of patients who have high expectations of being cured and who want to have a child.

We have learned that the advanced stage of cancers found in pregnancy are often due to delayed diagnosis (being hidden in the enlarged lactating breast) rather than to growth stimulation (see Chap. 16). We have learned that fertility is retained in a reasonable percentage (but not all) of younger patients who receive chemotherapy. Over the years, reports of pregnancies in small numbers of patients with breast cancer have appeared. None of the reports include more than 30 to 40 pregnancies in cohorts of several hundred young women with breast cancer. The reports do have a common theme. Except in those patients who conceived within 6 months of diagnosis, the recurrence rates and deaths from cancer were no higher among the pregnant patients than among matched controls, and, indeed, data suggest that the patients who had pregnancies 2 or more years after diagnosis may have done better than those who did not get pregnant.

In interpreting these studies, it must be remembered that there are thousands of fertile women who have had breast cancer, and we have no information at all about the numbers of pregnancies not brought to term. In addition, we do not know whether the absence of information about progressive disease with pregnancy means that it doesn't happen or that it is not reported. We must recognize that the patients who carried the pregnancies to term may have been preselected to be among the lower risk groups. Nevertheless, except in that early pregnancy group, there is no suggestion of significant worsening of prognosis.

Certainly no one would recommend term pregnancy in women receiving chemotherapy or hormonal therapy—the risk of fetal malformation is too high.

However, once therapy is completed, it is reasonable to consider the possibility. As with everything in medicine, we must weigh the risk and the cost against the potential benefit. And we must remember to include consideration of the risks, benefits, and future welfare of the child in our discussion.

A patient who has had a large aggressive tumor, with multiple positive nodes, has a high risk of recurrence. If the disease recurs, it will be incurable. If this woman has a child, there is a 50% to 60% chance that she will not live to see the child raised. She should be counseled regarding the trauma the child will experience by her death, and on the future care and well-being of the child.

A patient who has had a small, nonaggressive tumor (see Chap. 15 for a discussion of risk of recurrence) may have a 90% chance of survival and may be a much better overall candidate for term pregnancy, with reasonable assurance that the welfare of both mother and child are protected. Once 2 or 3 years have passed and no sign of recurrence has appeared, pregnancy may be considered.

Suggested Reading

Osteoporosis

Dalsky GP, et al. Weight-bearing exercise training and lumbar bone mineral content in postmenopausal women. *Ann Intern Med* 108: 824–828, 1988.

Riggs BL, and Melton LJ. The prevention and treatment of osteoporosis. *N Engl J Med* 327:620–627, 1992.

Pregnancy

Danforth DN. How subsequent pregnancy affects outcome in women with a prior breast cancer. *Oncol* 5:23–29, 1991.

Hassey KM. Pregnancy and parenthood after treatment for breast cancer. *Oncol Nurs Forum* 15:439–444, 1988.

Sutton R, Buzdar AU, and Hortobagyi G. Pregnancy and offspring after adjuvant chemotherapy in breast cancer patients. *Cancer* 65: 847–850, 1990.

Radiation Therapy

Boyce JD, et al. Cancer in the contralateral breast after radiotherapy for breast cancer. *N Engl J Med* 326:781–785, 1992.

Recht A, et al. Conservative surgery and radiation therapy for early breast cancer: Results, controversies and unsolved problems. *Sem Oncol* 13:434–449, 1986.

Wazer DE, et al. Factors influencing cosmetic outcome and complication risk after conservative surgery and radiotherapy for early-stage breast carcinoma. *J Clin Oncol* 10:356–363, 1992.

Chemotherapy

Curtis RE, et al. Risk of leukemia after chemotherapy and radiation treatment for breast cancer. *N Engl J Med* 326:1745–1751, 1992.

Myers SE, and Schilsky RL. Prospects for fertility after cancer chemotherapy. *Sem Oncol* 19:597–604, 1992.

Perry MC. Toxicity: Ten Years Later. *Sem Oncol* 19:453–457, 1992.

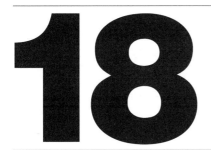

Follow-Up After Breast Cancer Treatment

Lois F. O'Grady

This chapter discusses recommendations for follow-up of patients treated for benign or malignant breast disease or both. The frequency of physician visits and the value of laboratory tests are considered.

Benign Disease

Symptomatic breast disease, for example, mastalgia, is often treated with hormonal manipulation. The resulting alterations in the pituitary-gonadal axis frequently lead to menstrual irregularities and other significant symptoms. When a course of hormonal therapy has been successful, it is prudent to schedule a follow-up visit 3 to 4 months later to assess whether symptoms have truly resolved and whether basic physiologic functioning has returned. The patient needs to be made aware that the disease tends to recur, and she should be encouraged to return if and when symptoms are bothersome.

Although a tissue diagnosis of benign breast disease is reassuring to both the patient and physician, a basic caveat must be remembered: *Any focal abnormality in the breast must be confirmed as benign or must be removed, and, except for simple cysts, must not recur or change.* This is especially important if the benign diagnosis is based on fine needle aspiration of a solid mass, which samples only portions of lesions. If a cyst keeps recurring, careful palpation of the area should be made after aspiration, and if a mass is suspected, a biopsy is necessary. If a palpable mass enlarges, a biopsy must be done to rule out the possibility that an underlying malignancy may be causing or affecting the abnormality.

It is important, therefore, that 3 months after a benign condition is diagnosed, a follow-up visit is scheduled to confirm that the breast remains normal or unchanged. For medicolegal purposes, it is mandatory that the physician's notes clearly document this scheduled return visit.

If a surgical biopsy has been done and the pathology report reveals truly benign conditions, such as fat necrosis, cystic changes, or mild, typical proliferative changes, then the patient may be followed according to routine guidelines, that is, with frequent breast self-

Table 18-1. Follow-up of benign breast disease

Follow-up visit 3 months after FNA or surgical biopsy
Regular breast self-examination
Yearly physical examination
Regular screening mammography*

*See Chap. 4 for mammography screening guidelines.
FNA = fine needle aspiration.

Table 18-2. Follow-up for high-risk patients

Follow-up visit 3 months after biopsy
Regular breast self-examination strongly encouraged and reinforced
Physical examination every 4 to 6 months
Rigorous adherence to mammography screening schedule*

*See Chaps. 4 and 12.

examination, yearly physical examination, and regularly scheduled mammography (Table 18-1).

However, if the biopsy reveals atypical hyperplasia or lobular carcinoma in situ, then the patient should be reclassified immediately as a patient with a definite increased risk of developing breast cancer. Breast self-examination should be strongly reinforced, physician examination should increase to every 4 to 6 months, and rigorous adherence to mammography guidelines should be instituted (Table 18-2).

Malignant Disease

The diagnosis of a malignant lesion in the breast initiates an intensive round of physician visits for treatment of the primary lesion. If adjuvant therapy is administered, the frequent visits may go on for 6 months. Unfortunately, once the frequency of visits decreases, patients may experience increased anxiety and depression resulting from the withdrawal of treatment ("My cancer isn't being treated anymore!") and the withdrawal of the significant support that had been provided by the physician and nursing staff every week or two. As the frequent visits end, the follow-up schedule should be explained so that the patient will understand what lies ahead and not feel as though she is being abandoned.

The oncologist and the referring physician should decide which of them will assume responsibility for the follow-up (it can be either), and this decision needs to be communicated clearly to the patient. She should be provided with a contact person with whom she may discuss symptoms or concerns and it should be made clear that she may schedule a return visit at any time.

It is helpful to give the patient a short list of what to watch out for (Table 18-3) and to remind her that just because she has cancer

Table 18-3. Symptoms and signs of recurrence

Thickenings, "pimples," or other skin changes near the scar
Lumps on the chest, above the clavicle, or under the arm
New, persistent bone pain of unknown etiology
Change in energy, appetite, or well-being
Cough or shortness of breath
Right upper quadrant discomfort, fullness, or pain

she is not immune to the aches and pains of daily life. Instruction on health maintenance, nutrition, and exercise should be provided as should encouragement to lead a normal life. Presumably, she underwent treatments so that she could enjoy life and she should be encouraged to do so.

Regularly scheduled office visits should be adhered to. These visits should address the topics listed under Components of Follow-Up and should *provide the patient adequate time to discuss her concerns.*

In the not too distant past, it was considered mandatory for all breast cancer patients to obtain frequent chest x-rays as well as yearly bone and liver scans. We now have data from many studies that suggest that these scans are unnecessary. In one large study, 74% of recurrences were found on history and examination; 36% were heralded by symptoms, 18% were found on patient self-examination, and 20% were discovered by physician examination. Another 12% of the recurrences were detected by chemistry panels, totaling 86%. Current thinking in oncology circles is that careful history and examination, and perhaps routine chemistry panels, are the mainstays of patient follow-up, along with the yearly mammogram. We also now have reasonable knowledge to predict which patients are at high risk for recurrence (e.g., those with large tumors, many positive lymph nodes, negative hormone receptors, and high S-phase [see Chap. 15]) and can target our health care dollars where they will do the most good. These philosophies are reflected in the recommendations that follow.

One must remember that well over 50% of these patients are cured of their breast cancer. They are not immune to other cancers or to other diseases and thus should not be denied regular health maintenance procedures (e.g., yearly Pap smear, mammogram of other breast, screening for colon cancer).

Components of Follow-Up

History
The schedule for patient follow-up visits is shown in Table 18-4. The history and review of systems should address the patient's general well-being and energy level. Has she resumed her regular schedule? Is she socializing as much as she used to? If she is single, is she dating? Have she and her partner made adequate adjustments sex-

Table 18-4. Schedule for follow-up visits*

Time	Low risk	High risk
Year 1	Every 3 months	Every 3 months
Years 2–5	Every 6 months	Every 4 months
Years 5–10	Yearly	Every 6 months
Years 10+	Yearly	Yearly

*History and physical examination should be done at each visit.

ually? Is she sleeping and eating as usual. How does *she* feel that she is adjusting?

Is she doing breast self-examination? If not, review it with her. Do her arm and shoulder have a full and easy range of motion? If not, refer her to a physical therapist.

Is she having any pain or discomfort? Is there any bone pain? If so, a bone scan, which shows changes long before they appear on x-ray, should be considered.

Is there any right upper quadrant discomfort? If so, a chemistry panel or a liver scan may be indicated.

Physical Examination
Vital signs are always important. Weight change can signal depression or discontent with body image (see Chap. 19). While taking the history, look for any signs of depression such as a flat affect or tears.

Examine the skin of the chest wall for signs of excessive thickening or fibrosis from radiation. Run the palm of your hand across the anterior and lateral chest wall. Because the typical subcutaneous nodularity can be felt before the recurrence can be seen, this is the best way to detect skin recurrences.

Examine the supraclavicular and axillary areas for nodes or recurrent tumor. The most effective way to examine the supraclavicular area is from behind. The axilla is best examined by standing in front of the patient and having her place her arm on your shoulder to let the weight of the arm fall on your shoulder. This relaxes the muscles around the axillae and provides the examining hand with easy access to the highest parts of the axillae. The fingers should sweep from the top down and any nodes will be felt passing between the fingers and the rib cage.

The breast(s) should be examined carefully, first with the patient in the sitting position and then again when she is recumbent with her arm(s) over her head to stretch the breast across the chest wall (see Figs. 7-1 and 7-2).

The lungs and liver should be checked as should other areas indicated by the review of systems.

Laboratory Studies
A complete blood count (CBC) and chemistry panels should be checked as outlined in Table 18-5.

Table 18-5. Schedule for laboratory tests

Test	Time	Low risk	High risk
CBC	Every 3 months until stable from chemotherapy, then yearly		
Chemistry panel	Years 0–5	Every 6 months	Each visit
	Years 5+	Yearly	Each visit
Serum markers*	Years 0–5	Every 6 months*	Every 6 months
	Years 5+	Yearly	Yearly

*May not be indicated (see text).

No serum marker for recurrent breast cancer is available that is as reliable as the carcinoembryonic antigen (CEA) for colon cancer and the prostate specific antigen (PSA) for prostate cancer. The best serum marker available for breast cancer is the cancer antigen 15-3 (CA 15-3), an antigen shed from the surface of most breast cancer cells. It is more frequently abnormal than any other marker, including the CEA. It is abnormal, however, in only 10% to 15% of patients with early breast cancer (stage I), 20% to 50% of patients with stage II disease, and 70% to 90% of patients with stage IV or metastatic disease. It is an excellent tool for following responses to therapy but is of limited value as a routine screening test for recurrence. Many oncologists order it regularly only in patients at high risk of recurrence or to help in the evaluation of suspected recurrences.

Radiologic Studies

A recommended schedule for radiologic testing is shown in Table 18-6. There is firm and documented evidence that routine mammography is essential in patients with breast cancer because a patient with one breast cancer carries a 20% lifetime risk (1% per year to the maximum of 20%) of developing a second breast cancer.

If the patient has undergone lumpectomy with radiation therapy or lumpectomy alone, for malignant disease, a new baseline mammogram, on the treatment side only, should be obtained when treatment is complete and the patient can tolerate the compression required for good quality films. This should be done within 6 months

Table 18-6. Schedule for radiologic studies

Study	Time	Low risk	High risk
Chest x-ray[a]	Years 0–5	Yearly	Yearly
	Years 5+	—	—
Mammography	—	Yearly	Yearly
Liver and bone scans[b]	Only if symptoms	Only if symptoms	Only if symptoms

[a]May not be indicated (see text).
[b]For very high-risk patients, some advocate that a baseline bone scan be done at diagnosis and then yearly to year 5. We do not agree.

of the lumpectomy. The reason is that scarring and postoperative distortion (Fig. 18-1) can be confused with recurrent cancer. The new baseline mammogram provides a reference against which one can detect architectural changes that may herald recurrent cancer. Any abnormality seen in a film taken within 6 months of therapy is most likely due to postsurgical scarring; the likelihood of recurrent cancer being present at this time is extremely small. The regular schedule of yearly bilateral mammography should be resumed 1 year after surgery.

There is no clear-cut evidence to indicate that any other radiologic procedure should be performed regularly. Regular chest x-rays (as shown on the schedules below) have become a habit; however, their

Fig. 18-1. Postsurgical scar. Right mediolateral mammogram showing a spiculated scar (*arrow*) from a previous lumpectomy for carcinoma. The scar is indistinguishable from a malignant lesion, but is in the location of the previous cancer and has remained stable for 7 years.

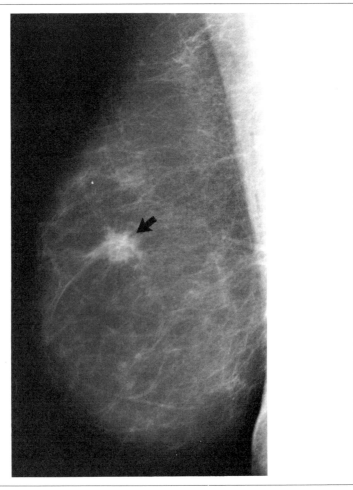

cost-effectiveness in patients in whom there is a low risk of recurrence is questionable, and many oncologists order routine chest x-rays only in patients at high risk of recurrence. At the same time one should recognize that many patients expect regular chest x-rays and may believe adequate care is not being provided if x-rays are not ordered. Here, the art of medicine must enter the decision arena.

There is evidence that routine liver and bone scanning is not cost-effective. A bone lesion as the first manifestation of recurrence occurs in less than 1% of patients, and, more important, almost invariably the patient becomes symptomatic within a short time of the positive bone scan. The difference in time is meaningless in the long-term management of the disease. Routine liver scanning is not cost-effective either because many liver recurrences are heralded by abnormalities in the chemistry panels or by the patient's symptoms. Sadly, a 1- or 2-month delay in documenting liver metastases makes little difference in the long run. In addition to the dollar cost of an unnecessary test, there is tremendous psychological cost to the patient in agonizing over the tests and waiting for results. To add needless stress to these patients is cruel.

Schedule of Follow-Up

Table 18-4 provides the recommended schedules for follow-up visits. High- and low-risk patients are defined by the criteria outlined in Chap. 15, the most important of which are tumor size and nodal status.

Special Considerations

A large number of patients with breast cancer are maintained on *tamoxifen* to prevent recurrence and to decrease the risk of second breast cancers (see Chap. 15). Although tamoxifen is a well-tolerated drug physicians must be aware of three potentially problematic areas.

First, there is a small but measurable increase in thromboembolic disease, such as there is with the oral contraceptives. Unilateral leg swelling, chest pain, or shortness of breath may need assessment with Doppler flow studies or scans.

Second, there may be gynecologic disturbances. About 6% of patients develop a mild vaginal discharge that is usually clear and watery. No concern need exist about this, and patients can be reassured that it does not represent disease. About 6% of patients develop vaginal dryness and may require lubricants during intercourse. In patients who have been on the drug for a long time there may be endometrial hyperplasia, which may progress to endometrial cancer in some patients. The incidence of endometrial cancer from tamoxifen use is about the same as that seen in women taking unopposed estrogen for postmenopausal symptoms, that is, about 1%

after 5 years. This is not a concern in women without a uterus or in those who continue to menstruate while receiving tamoxifen because the uterus lining sloughs regularly. In other patients, abnormal vaginal bleeding should be investigated promptly with endometrial biopsies. Some physicians recommend routine endometrial biopsies for all patients on long-term tamoxifen, but most physicians feel this is excessive, overreactive, not cost-effective, and thus should not be done. Patients tend to agree. A more prudent approach is yearly pelvic examination with Pap smear. After 3 years the thickness of the uterine lining can be assessed with transvaginal ultrasonography. If the uterine lining is >4 mm in thickness, curettage or biopsy can be considered to determine whether endometrial dysplasia is present. If so, one should consider discontinuing tamoxifen.

The third problem to be aware of is hot flashes. As is true with regular menopausal patients, the frequency and severity of flashes vary from patient to patient, and bother some more than others. For those bothered mostly at night, the antihistamine diphenhydramine (25–50 mg) sometimes controls the flashes so that the patient can get a good night's sleep. For patients in whom diphenhydramine is ineffective or for those whose hot flashes are most bothersome in the daytime, Bellergal-S (a complex of phenobarbital, ergotamine, and belladonna) may be helpful. The usual dosage is one tablet in the morning and one at night, but some do not like the side effects, which include dry mouth, blurred vision, and drowsiness. Finally, clonidine controls the symptoms in some patients. It can be given in a pill form (0.1 mg once or twice a day), or in a transdermal preparation (0.1 mg every 5–7 days), starting with the lowest dose and escalating as tolerated.

General Health Measures

Women with breast cancer have an increased risk of developing other tumors, of the breast, of course, but also of gynecologic and colonic tumors. Annual pelvic examinations with Pap smears are advised for all women. For women over 50 years of age, testing for occult blood in the stool and rectal examinations should be routine.

Most patients with breast cancer must spend several years without endogenous or exogenous estrogen, because of the fear that estrogen may stimulate the growth of residual cancer cells and contribute to the development of second primary cancers (see Chap. 12 regarding antiestrogen prophylaxis of breast cancer and Chap. 10 on the estrogen-deprived patient). To prevent osteoporosis, a program of regular weight-bearing exercise and extra calcium is mandatory. Brisk walking for 40 minutes 3 to 4 times a week is the minimum and 1500 mg per day of calcium supplementation is recommended.

A well-balanced diet is prudent. There is some evidence, although it is becoming more tenuous with time, that excess animal fat in the diet may be linked to the induction of cancer; thus, a diet low in animal fat is recommended by nutrition experts (see Chap. 3). There is much less evidence that it affects growth of cancer already present. Patients should be warned against fad anticancer diets, and of the dangers of excessive vitamin A and D, which are often advocated by practitioners of alternative medicine. Vitamin A is hepatotoxic in excessive amounts (synergistically toxic with alcohol and other hepatotoxins) and can cause abnormal liver function tests. Excessive vitamin D can cause hypercalcemia. Both are stored in fat and can be released in excessive and toxic amounts in the unfortunate patients who develop metastatic disease and become bedridden and malnourished.

Suggested Reading

Epstein AH, et al. The predictors of distant relapse following conservative surgery and radiotherapy for early breast cancer are similar to those following mastectomy. *Int J Rad Oncol Biol Phys* 17: 755–760, 1989.

Logager VB, et al. The limited value of routine chest x-ray in the follow-up of stage II breast cancer. *Eur J Cancer* 26:553–555, 1990.

Loomer L, et al. Postoperative follow-up of patients with early breast cancer. *Cancer* 67:55–60, 1991.

Moskovic E, Parsons C, and Baum M. Chest radiography in the management of breast cancer. *Br J Radiol* 65:30–32, 1992.

Pandya KJ, et al. A retrospective study of earliest indicators of recurrence in patients on eastern cooperative oncology group adjuvant chemotherapy trials for breast cancer. *Cancer* 55:202–205, 1985.

Tondini C, Hayes DF, and Kufe DW. Circulating tumor markers in breast cancer. *Hematol Oncol Clin North Am* 3:653–674, 1989.

Wickerhan L, Fisher B, Cronin W, and Members of the NSABP Committee for Treatment Failure Criteria. The efficacy of bone scanning in the follow-up of patients with operable breast cancer. *Breast Cancer Res Treat* 4:303–307, 1984.

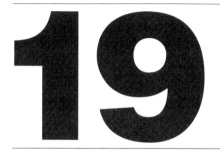

Restoration of Body Image After Mastectomy

Linda Clemence Reib,
Lois F. O'Grady,
and Debra A. Reilly

For some women, restoration of body image after mastectomy is simply a matter of altering their psychological perception of "self." Some women view themselves in terms of their accomplishments in life, their security in their lifestyle, or their grounding in religion. For other women their physical body image is a major force behind self-image, and for a few women body image is the dominating factor in their self-esteem and self-confidence. Dealing with a threat to a component of one's self-esteem can be staggering even for the most self-assured woman.

Establishing good communication between a woman and her physician plays a vital role in helping the patient understand her options following a mastectomy. Some women will choose breast reconstruction. Some may undergo this surgery immediately, others may choose to wait, and some will never explore this option.

The recovery process can be made easier even while a woman is still in the hospital. The American Cancer Society's Reach to Recovery program is an effective way for a woman to see the positive results of a life after a mastectomy and to see that the crisis of breast cancer can be mastered. Reach to Recovery is staffed by female volunteers, all of whom have been carefully selected and trained. These women have all had breast cancer and have fully adjusted to their surgery. Volunteers, who have taken it upon themselves to openly share their experiences with other women, will visit a breast cancer patient while she is in the hospital. Upon a doctor's referral, a patient will be introduced to the realities of her breast loss. She will be provided a kit that includes a soft, comfortable filler for her bra, so that she may leave the hospital looking natural. Information on exercises to restore full range of motion to the arm on the affected side and lists of where to buy prostheses, bras, and swimwear are also included. The volunteers are sympathetic and comforting, having been through this experience themselves. A woman who has just had her breast removed may be curious to see what other chest walls look like. Reach to Recover volunteers have been known to reveal their own surgery and to provide the patient her first look at a breast prosthesis. This experience can be rewarding and can be the first step toward a positive, healthy rehabilitation.

If there is no American Cancer Society office in your area, check with the local YWCA, church council, or hospital. Recognizing the vital role that support plays in a faster recovery, many lay groups have developed counseling programs. National organizations, listed in Appendix C, may have information on local support groups.

In order to restore her body image after mastectomy, a patient has two options—reconstruction or use of a prosthesis.

Reconstructive Surgery

Breast reconstruction is now commonly performed after mastectomy. There are various types of operations available (see below) and virtually no restrictions on when the procedures should be performed.

It is important for the patient to understand that there are no operations available that recreate a perfect breast in one operation. Usually a breast "mound" is created to match the aesthetics of the opposite breast, and frequently this requires one or two other minor procedures to achieve symmetry. An additional procedure will be needed if the recreation of a nipple-areolar complex is desired.

Deciding on the timing of the reconstructive procedure should involve a dialogue between patient, surgeon, reconstructive surgeon, and medical oncologist. Optimally, a separate preoperative consultation with the reconstructive surgeon is held.

Immediate Reconstruction

Immediate reconstruction is performed during the same anesthetic as the ablative procedure. Advantages of immediate reconstruction are that the patient usually does not require a second hospital admission (secondary reconstructive procedures are frequently done on an outpatient basis), only one anesthetic is required, and the patient awakens from her mastectomy without the total absence of a breast mound and thus may not experience a staggering sense of loss.

Disadvantages of immediate reconstruction include prolonged anesthetic time, potential for blood loss requiring blood transfusions, a slightly higher minor complication rate, and the possibility of a delay in starting adjuvant therapy (radiation or chemotherapy) if a complication from the reconstructive procedure occurs.

Delayed Reconstruction

Delayed reconstruction implies that the patient has undergone definitive cancer surgery with or without adjuvant therapy. The stage of her disease is now known, and adjuvant therapies, if needed, can be given. The toxicities of the adjuvant therapies may interfere with wound healing or, conversely, a wound complication may delay a necessary adjuvant therapy. It is best to begin the reconstructive process after local therapy is completed. Reconstruction can start once the adjuvant therapy is completed when blood counts have returned to normal and local skin reaction from radiation has subsided, or any time thereafter.

The advantage of delayed reconstruction is that it gives the patient time—time for psychosocial adjustment, time to complete adjuvant therapy, and time to explore the use of prosthetic devices as an alternative to reconstruction.

Contraindications

An advanced local stage of breast cancer is a relative but not an absolute contraindication to a reconstructive procedure. The patient should not have ongoing, active disease for which she is undergoing radiotherapy or chemotherapy. Patients with metastatic disease are not good candidates for reconstruction because of their limited survival. Associated medical conditions that may increase the risk of anesthesia or surgery are relative contraindications to reconstructive surgery.

Autologous Tissue Versus Implant Reconstruction

Autologous tissue or synthetic implants can be used to create a breast. The procedure selected by the plastic surgeon and patient depends, in part, on anatomic considerations, the size of the breast to be created, and the general health status and lifestyle of the patient. Table 19-1 outlines the advantages, disadvantages, and contraindications of implant-use versus autologous-tissue reconstruction.

Autologous Tissue

The use of autologous tissue involves transfer of composite tissue from other areas of the patient's body to the mastectomy site in order to recreate the natural breast mound. Myocutaneous flaps are advantageous because the muscle receives its blood supply from a dominant artery and the overlying skin and subcutaneous tissues are fed from the same arterial system. Suitable donor tissues include the latissimus dorsi myocutaneous flap, the transverse rectus abdominus myocutaneous (TRAM) flap, the lateral thigh fasciocutaneous flap, and the gluteus myocutaneous flap. The first two can be transferred as local tissue (pedicle flaps) while they all may be transferred as free flaps. Bilateral breasts can be reconstructed using bilateral flaps in one or two staged procedures.

Each of these procedures allows a breast mound to be created at the time of the first operation as part of the mastectomy, or later. Figure 19-1 shows a patient shortly after a TRAM flap has been used to create a breast mound. Note that the ptotic effect approximates that of the normal breast, an effect difficult to achieve with implants. One or two small outpatient procedures to tailor the flaps are necessary to obtain an aesthetically pleasing result. If inadequate soft

Table 19-1. Comparison of three reconstructive procedures

Procedure	Advantages	Disadvantages	Contraindications
Tissue expansion, implant	Simple Outpatient surgery Existing breast scar used	Foreign body Bra cup size limited	Excessive postradiation fibrosis Intolerance to silicone
Latissimus dorsi myocutaneous flap	No foreign body Less surgery than TRAM Hearty, viable flap	Bra cup limited to B or C Shoulder girdle impaired Visible scar results	Professional athletics Smoking Denervation from mastectomy
TRAM flap	No foreign body More tissue Scar better concealed Tummy tuck Good skin-texture results	Most surgery Potential increase in blood loss Abdominal muscles impaired	Professional athletics Smoking Obesity Previous abdominal surgery

TRAM = transverse rectus abdominus myocutaneous.

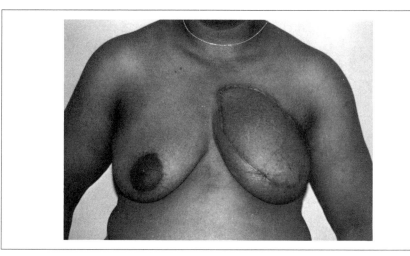

Fig. 19-1. A patient is shown shortly after surgery in which a TRAM flap has been used to create a breast mound.

tissue is available the patient may elect to have a breast implant placed beneath her flap tissue. Generally, some time is allowed for the flap to settle before the nipple-areolar complex reconstruction is started; many women do not desire nipple-areolar reconstruction and elect to do without nipples or to use paste-on nipples instead.

If a nipple-areolar complex is to be created, tissue can be obtained from behind the ear, from the inner thigh, or from the inferior gluteal crease and transferred as skin grafts to form the areolar. The nipple is formed either from local tissue or by transferring tissue from the opposite nipple. Simple surgical tattooing of an areola is sufficient for a small percentage of patients.

Multiple factors affect the choice of a flap. For example, a professional golfer, tennis player, or swimmer may not want the latissimus muscle moved while a gymnast might not want the loss of abdominal musculature resulting from a TRAM flap. Some women may not want the additional visible scar on the back from the latissimus flap; others may want the tummy tuck of the TRAM flap procedure. Only a TRAM flap provides enough tissue to create a larger breast, but a woman who smokes is not a good candidate for any myocutaneous flap, especially a TRAM flap, because of potential vascular problems. An obese woman is more likely to get abdominal hernias following rectus muscle transfers.

Implant Reconstruction

A breast mound can be created using an implant, as shown in Fig. 19-2. Implants can be placed in the subpectoral position in a size large enough to match the opposite breast. Unfortunately, because of the loss of the overlying soft tissue that results from the ablative procedure, not enough skin remains to simply elevate the flaps and

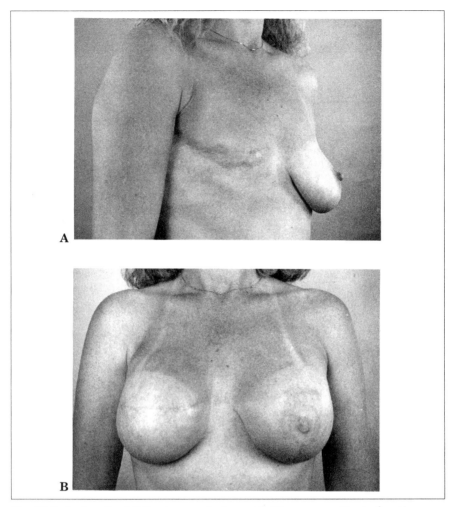

Fig. 19-2. A. A patient following mastectomy. B. The same patient after tissue expansion and implant placement on the right and mastopexy on the left.

to place an implant in the manner in which an augmentation mammaplasty is performed. Instead, a staged reconstructive plan is followed, which begins by first placing a tissue expander underneath the muscle and serially (weekly) injecting fluid into the expander to stretch the overlying soft tissues. Expansion is carried out to a size slightly larger than the opposite breast and maintained at this volume for several weeks to months until the flaps are soft. At this time, the expander is deflated, removed, and replaced with a permanent breast implant. The FDA now has approved the placement of silicone shell/gel-filled implants only if the patient and surgeon are participating in an FDA-approved safety and efficacy study. Otherwise, a silicone shell/saline-filled implant is used. This exchange of the expander for the implant is usually performed as an outpatient procedure and may be done in conjunction with the re-creation of the nipple-areolar complex.

Disadvantages and potential complications of implants are discussed in Chap. 11. Other disadvantages to this method of reconstruction include the need for weekly visits to have the expander inflated and the potential embarrassment of having one's breast size and shape change weekly during the expansion process. In addition, in attempting to match a very large breast, there may be a practical limit to the size of the implant to be inserted. In this case, autologous tissue may be required for the reconstructed breast or the normal breast may need to be reduced.

Advantages of implant reconstruction are the relatively simple procedures, the generally short hospital stay, and the lack of interference with adjuvant chemotherapy.

The aesthetics of the opposite breast are often addressed by the plastic surgeon at the time of breast reconstruction. An exceptionally large breast can be reduced or a droopy, ptotic breast can be lifted by mastopexy. Occasionally, a patient may choose to have a larger breast profile and may have her native breast augmented to match a larger reconstructed breast.

Prostheses

For those women who choose to avoid reconstruction either temporarily or permanently, the physician should stress the importance of a properly fitted breast form, one that is weighted and that will help restore balance and symmetry to the chest wall. Physicians should be sensitive to the importance of figure enhancement and a natural appearance, because these are vital for regaining feelings of femininity and self-assurance in most patients.

Each woman who elects to investigate the purchase of a breast prosthesis makes the transition from patient to consumer. The remainder of this chapter assists the physician in educating the patient to become an informed consumer on postmastectomy products.

A positive starting point is the American Cancer Society's breast form display. This is a presentation of breast forms, swimwear, wigs, and all items that may be needed following breast surgery and adjuvant therapy. The display is staffed by volunteers who offer information and answer questions in a relaxed atmosphere. Call your local American Cancer Society office for times and dates.

Facilities

Most women are ready for an initial fitting of a breast prosthesis within 4 to 6 weeks of surgery. Clearance from the physician is required because healing times vary. There are some women who will wait a year or more simply because a prosthesis was not discussed with them. A prescription is required for insurance coverage.

Not all communities offer a choice of facilities that carry postmastectomy products. Large metropolitan areas may offer several boutiques that specialize in breast forms and related apparel. Specialty stores are superior to department stores in that they offer personalized service, a greater selection of products, and specially trained personnel. Other resources for the patient are home health care suppliers, mail order catalogs, major department stores, medical supply houses, orthotic and prosthetic facilities, and pharmacies.

If a variety of facilities are available, certain criteria can help the patient select the most suitable:

1. Does the supplier have certified fitters on staff? These individuals have been given extensive training by the surgical supply companies on the product as well as on measuring techniques, anatomy, and the various types of surgical procedures.
2. Is the facility warm and receptive in appearance?
3. Does the facility have private fitting rooms with adequate lighting?
4. Are a large variety of shapes, sizes, brands, and bras available?
5. Is insurance billing acceptable?

The Fitting

A pleasant, comfortable atmosphere is vital to foster a positive experience for the postmastectomy woman. Most important is a fitter who is friendly, compassionate, and professional and whose nonverbal communication immediately puts the woman at ease. For the majority of women, this is the first time they have shown their chest wall to nonmedical personnel and perhaps their first confrontation with a mirror. An experienced fitter will take the time necessary to establish a relationship with the customer, to discuss her lifestyle and expectations regarding her prosthesis, and to encourage and answer any questions.

The fitting consists of selecting the correct bra and the proper prosthesis. It is helpful for the woman to bring to the fitting a sample of her favorite style of bra, a striped T-shirt and a front-buttoning blouse, a swimsuit, and her husband, friend, or other support person.

The woman should expect to spend at least 30 minutes in the fitting room, trying on several different styles of bras and prostheses of various shapes and weights. When she leaves she should be aware that she will need some time to get used to the prosthesis and that a more firm bra may be more comfortable once the swelling and tenderness have disappeared. She should have a guarantee from the facility that they will take care of her needs if the fit is not comfortable.

The Prosthesis

Over the years, breast prostheses have evolved to accommodate various techniques, from the Halsted radical mastectomy to the modified radical mastectomy to the quadrantectomy. The basic objective of all prostheses is to replace the volume of lost breast tissue necessary to achieve skeletal balance as well as proper external contour.

Stock or preformed breast forms are available in sizes 28AA to 50FF and in a variety of shapes and skin tones as seen in Fig. 19-3. They are generally guaranteed for 2 years. Custom prostheses can be cast to fit and match any chest wall. Both preformed and custom prostheses are available in various skin tones.

Most women replace their breast form every 2 to 4 years. Replacement should be encouraged because weight changes, body habitus changes, and other medical conditions may arise requiring a different style, shape, or weight of prosthesis.

Newer surgical techniques for mastectomies and changing fashion modes have dictated the need for breast forms that are soft and natural in appearance. Most manufacturers meet that need by using silicone to produce the most functional, reliable, and comfortable product. The silicone is encased in a hypoallergenic polyurethane envelope and is appropriately weighted to match the remaining breast. Soft and almost realistic to the touch, semisolid silicone forms do not leak or absorb moisture, making them ideal for the active woman.

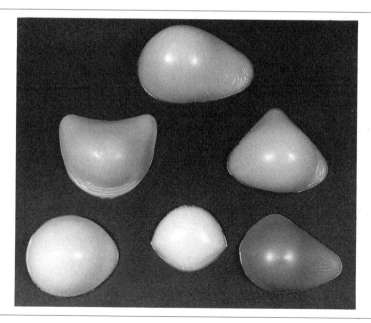

Fig. 19-3. A small sample of the variety of sizes, shapes, and colors of breast prostheses.

Other possible materials include sculpted foam, for a lighter weight prosthesis, and a liquid-filled form, which is more cost-effective. Leisure breast forms consist of a poly-fiberfill. These lightweight forms tend to ride high on the chest wall, increasing the risk of neck, shoulder, and back aches from skeletal imbalance. We recommend, therefore, that these leisure breast forms be worn at nighttime only.

All of the other breast forms are designed to be worn daily, during all activities. The new attachment system with which the prosthesis adheres directly to the skin (Fig. 19-4) can be worn while bathing and swimming; the silicone is safe in hot tubs, pools, and saunas. All breast forms should be gently washed as needed with mild soap and water, allowed to air dry, and kept in the original custom-molded container.

Bras

With the exception of the attachment system and custom-made products, all prostheses are worn inside a bra. The forms are inserted into a pocket, which has been sewn into the bra and which offers security. The pocket, usually of soft cotton, provides an absorbent layer between the breast form and the skin.

Determining the correct bra size is basic to the selection process. The bra may be soft cup or underwire. Depending on specific anatomic considerations, it can have wider straps for increased support and less tension on the shoulder, a deeper underband to keep the bra from riding up onto the incision, and posterior strap adjustments for a nonbinding fit and to prevent the clasp from chafing the anterior chest wall. Regardless of the structural changes required in the garment, the product is still attractive, as shown in Fig. 19-5.

Clothing and Swimwear

Most women require few changes in wardrobe with a prosthesis. However, special circumstances may necessitate adjustments and a variety of products are thus available: for example, looser sleeves (if lymphedema develops), specially designed swimwear with slightly higher neck and underarm lines (to cover scars), and lingerie designed with pockets to hold the prosthesis (so she doesn't have to wear a bra to bed).

Fig. 19-4. A soft, pliable adhesive-backed prosthesis faced with hook and loop material (A) can attach to matching strips adherent to the chest wall (B and C). No bra is required, and the strips will stay in place for several days. (Courtesy of Amoena Corporation.)

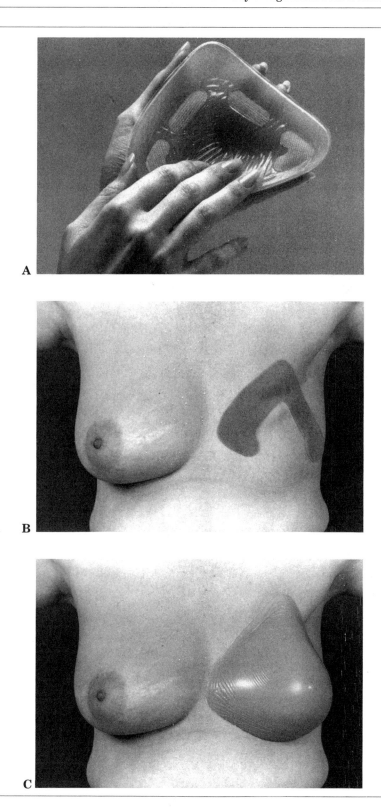

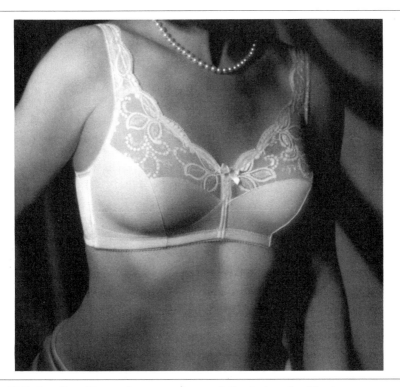

Fig. 19-5. An attractive undergarment especially designed with strap adjustments in the back and wider shoulder straps. It contains a pocket on the left to hold a prosthesis. (Courtesy of Amoena Corporation.)

Insurance

Many women struggle with the decision to invest in a well-fitted bra and prosthesis. It is, however, one of the most important purchases she can make and a critical part in the restoration of her self-assurance. It is definitely the time to be a little free with money. The burden of cost can be softened by the fact that most insurance companies cover breast forms and bras. As soon as the incisions have healed, advise the patient to get a prosthesis and provide her with a prescription that includes the following information:

1. Breast prosthesis (left, right, or bilateral) with mastectomy bra
2. Diagnosis
3. Date of surgery
4. License number and other identification required by state or federal law.

Financial coverage will vary according to individual policies and some policies may require prior authorization. Medicare coverage provides for breast forms and bras. Reimbursement differs geographically, but payment will usually be (unless federally mandated) 80% of the allowable.

Women without insurance need not go without a prosthesis. Their options include Medicaid, donated forms from the American Cancer Society, county programs through social services, and local churches and support groups.

Lymphedema

Although lymphedema occurs less often with the more modern surgical and radiotherapy techniques now being used, some women do develop arm swelling. It is a disappointing complication and can negatively impact the patient's body image. Untreated, the affected limb increases in size and increases the risk of infection. Several modes of therapy have become available, the most common of which is the use of a sequential gradient compression pump. An inflatable sleeve is connected to an external pneumatic pump. Pressure is established from the distal area of the sleeve and progresses upward until the entire sleeve is sequentially inflated. When the sleeve is filled with air, the cells in the sleeve empty, and the cycle repeats. This cycle forces fluid centrally, "milking" the edema fluid and thus reducing swelling (see Appendix C for resource information).

When the arm is maximally reduced, the patient can be measured for a compression garment (a heavy elastic sleeve) to be worn during the day. Appendix C contains information on these pumps.

Manual lymph drainage, popular in Europe for years, is now becoming available in the United States. This method of massage, using the therapist's hands as a milking device, moves the stagnant fluid out of the affected limb (see Appendix C for resource information).

Suggested Reading

Bostwick J. Reconstruction after mastectomy. *Surg Clin North Am* 70:1125–1140, 1990.

Field DA, and Miller S. Cosmetic breast surgery. *Am Fam Phys* 45: 711–719, 1992.

Gross A, and Ito D. *Women Talk about Breast Surgery*. New York: Clarkson Potter, 1990.

Hang-Fu H, and Snyderman RK. State-of-the-art breast reconstruction. *Cancer* 68:1148–1156, 1991.

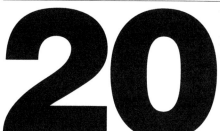

The Terminally Ill Patient

Mary E. Kennedy
and Lois F. O'Grady

Despite hopes to the contrary, a certain percentage of patients with breast cancer will die of their disease. In fact, the yearly mortality rate from breast cancer has not changed in the past 50 years. The increased number of cures from early detection and treatment has matched the increased incidence of the disease.

The diagnosis of metastatic disease is a fearful one for the patient and for the health care team because almost all of these women are incurable. There is treatment—judicious use of chemotherapy, radiation therapy, and surgery can prolong a comfortable, functional life for a few years. But the time comes when the patient and the oncologist recognize that the potential benefit of continuing anticancer therapies is outweighed by the loss of quality of life. The time at which this point is reached varies from patient to patient and from physician to physician. Some patients and physicians want to continue aggressive therapies until the last hope of benefit is exhausted, regardless of the quality of life. Others place quality of life ahead of quantity at an earlier time.

Unfortunately, some physicians have come to view chemotherapy and radiation therapy as the only interventions for the cancer patient and see stopping them as "giving up." Wise physicians know better and will have taken time during the course of treatment of the metastatic disease to establish open, honest communication with the patient and her family. Important discussions revolve around the issues of quantity versus quality of life, and the mutual establishment of therapeutic goals to prolong functional and comfortable life when possible and to alleviate pain and suffering at all times. The tools used to accomplish the goals will vary with time. Initially, chemotherapy and radiation might be part of the treatment plan, but at some point these will be replaced by therapeutic modalities geared more toward comfort. If this is done well, there is no sense of giving up, but rather a sense of changing focus to fit the changing needs of the patient.

Maintaining hope is crucial to the patient, her family, and her loved ones. During the process of adjusting to the knowledge that the disease is terminal, it is important for the physician to guide the patient and family in refocusing their hope. Some patients and families may express their fear that if hope for a cure is gone, there will be nothing to live for. However, quality of life, meaningful personal relationships, completion of unfinished business, and saying good-bye in a way that leaves the family and loved ones stronger are all worthy of hope.

When chemotherapy and radiation therapy are no longer being employed, the patient may choose to see the oncologist less often and the primary care physician more frequently. An honest and open dialogue among all concerned is mandatory to establish lines of responsibility, with the primary concern being the welfare of the patient. Some factors that enter into the decision involve the physician's level of comfort with care of the dying patient, the physician's association with a hospice program, the distance of the physician from the patient's home town, and the bonding of the patient and family with one physician or another.

Once the lines of responsibility are clearly defined, the entire focus is on palliative care. To accomplish this, referral to a hospice team may be appropriate. Although initially conceived as an inpatient facility for the dying, the concept of hospice has broadened significantly. Today, the goal is to provide physical, emotional, and spiritual support for terminally ill patients and their families, 24 hours a day, 7 days a week, in the home environment. To allow a patient to spend the last months of life in her own home, among her own memorabilia, sleeping in her own bed with her partner, and *remaining in control of her daily life,* is a valuable gift. All hospice teams have the same general requirements (Table 20-1). Individual programs may have additional criteria, depending on local resources and regulations. The hospice team includes a physician, who approves all treatment plans and is available for consultation, nurses specially trained in palliative care and pain management, social workers skilled in counseling, and home health aides who provide personal care and assist the family. Physical therapists and other health personnel can be incorporated as appropriate for an individual patient's needs. Many hospice teams include chaplains, bereavement counselors, and community volunteers.

With or without the assistance of a hospice team, care of the terminally ill addresses comfort, of mind as well as of body.

Comfort of Mind

Comfort of mind begins with the establishment of open, honest communication among all concerned: patient, family or other care givers, and the health care team. If the physician is not skilled in interpersonal communication, the responsibility should be delegated to someone who is—a social worker, nurse, or another individual. It is important for the patient to feel that her needs can be made known and her fears verbalized without jeopardizing care. Dying patients have two primary concerns—being abandoned by their physician

Table 20-1. General requirements for home hospice care

Diagnosis of terminal disease with life expectancy of 6 months or less.
Patient must be aware of the prognosis and give informed consent to a
   palliative plan of treatment.
Patient has a capable care giver (family, friend, or paid attendant) willing
   to accept responsibility.
The home environment is safe for the patient, care giver, and hospice
   staff.
The physician agrees to work with the hospice team.
Appropriate funding is available.

when it is apparent that they are dying and the fear of dying in
intractable pain.

Resuscitation or Code Status

The patient and family must be made aware that the patient has a
terminal disease, and the goals of palliative care need to be clearly
defined.

The discussion, ideally led by the physician in a quiet, comfortable
environment and without time constraints, should be with the
patient and whoever is going to hold her designated power of attorney for health care decisions. This discussion will prevent misinter-
pretations in the future. The physician should guide the discussion
appropriately. For example, asking the question "Do you want me to
do everything possible to keep you alive?" may elicit an inappropriate
response because the patient and physician may attach different
meanings to the word *everything*. Rephrasing it to "How do you feel
about the use of machines to keep cancer patients alive?" will often
bring about a more realistic response. A question like this provides
the patient an opportunity to verbalize her concerns and provides a
forum to discuss dignity in death. Encouraging the patient and
family to stay at home for the terminal phase of the disease avoids
many pitfalls and lessens the chance of inappropriate medical
interventions.

Cardiopulmonary resuscitation (CPR) has never cured cancer.
Studies have shown that functional survival after CPR in cancer
patients is extraordinarily rare and that it is a futile therapeutic
maneuver. This information must be communicated to the patient
and family, and if they agree, a "Do Not Resuscitate" (DNR) order
should be written prominently in the medical record. It is important
that the patient and family be told clearly that "no code" does not
mean "no care." A copy of the DNR order should be kept in a prominent place in the home, in case a well-meaning but misguided individual calls 911. Ambulance crews, in general, must attempt resuscitation and cannot accept verbal orders from the family or physician. It is also helpful to bring the DNR order with the patient

if she is transported to a hospital for a symptom-control procedure, such as thoracentesis or palliative radiation therapy.

Legal Issues

At some point attention must be given to legal matters: the drawing up of a will, the clear, legal delegation of responsibility for care of children, and the establishment of a durable power of attorney for health care. This is especially critical for single parents. Arrangements for another person to have power of attorney or other clear authority for financial decisions and access to the family finances is necessary. These matters should be addressed early on while the patient is clear of mind and competent to make legal and financial decisions. Once this is accomplished, patients often feel a great sense of relief.

Spiritual Issues

Death is a frightening concept for most people. Patients facing death usually seek spiritual guidance. For those who have had long-standing religious affiliations, pastoral care may have been a service provided from the beginning. For those who have not been closely linked to an organized religion, this is the time to ask whether the patient wishes to talk with a minister, priest, rabbi, or other religious figure. Hospice programs and hospital chaplains can provide spiritual support or can make the appropriate referrals.

Dying is inherently a spiritual crisis, but the discussion of spiritual matters in our culture is alien to many and a difficult subject to address for many more. Talking with the patient about funeral services or burial plans can open the door to conversations on spiritual matters.

Family Issues

It is a rare family that has no skeletons in the closet, no lingering animosity over almost-forgotten hurts, or no lost sheep. The end of life is a time for completion, a time for healing and forgiving. Unresolved issues of life naturally surface when a patient and her family speak freely of the impending death. Physicians should encourage their patients to complete unfinished relationships with loved ones and to seek the emotional support necessary to make this possible. Some patients and families are able to invite friends and loved ones to visit and to say good-bye, but most need the direction and support of a social worker, hospice team member, or clergy. Such visits provide peace of mind for the dying and lighten the grief for those who remain.

Even though one family member may be designated the primary care giver, all members of the family should be involved and given certain tasks to perform or responsibilities to fulfill. This approach gives everyone a sense of "doing something," fosters family unity and communication, and helps to alleviate guilt and remorse after the death. This is especially important if there are children in the home. Honesty is always the best policy with children. They should be made aware of what is happening and allowed to be part of the process. Knowing that they helped take care of Mother, that they gave her a valued gift, can be immensely helpful to children in dealing with their grief.

The patient should be given the opportunity to inform the family of her wishes regarding distribution of memorabilia, clothing, and favorite pieces of jewelry. Such discussions are healing and give the patient an opportunity to give someone a gift, a special remembrance; this giving brings pleasure and peace to the patient.

Personal Issues

Family members, particularly spouses, should allow the patient to discuss any aspect of their personal relationship. The physician, or other member of the health care team, can facilitate this openness by raising the issue as part of a quiet office or home visit. For example, a wife may want to give her husband permission to remarry. The husband should give his wife the opportunity to offer this gift. Such communications are part of anticipatory grief and allow the remaining partner to begin the bereavement process.

Comfort of Body

Serenity of mind is best achieved when the body is without stress. The patient's physical environment, general health status (including hydration and elimination), and pain control all contribute to bodily comfort.

Physical Environment

Initially, the patient may be fully ambulatory, needing little or no physical assistance. As the patient becomes more frail, ambulatory-assist devices such as canes, walkers, or wheelchairs are useful. Patients who can be out of bed, participating in family activities in the home and taking excursions out of the home, are happier and more content.

An electric hospital bed with trapeze, either in the bedroom or in a center of family activity, can help the patient move independently and makes it easier for the care giver. A portable commode is helpful for some patients.

It is important that the patient know that assistance is available at all times, but provision also must be made for privacy and solitude.

We all need a certain amount of "space" (some of us need more than others) and terminally ill patients are no exception. Most patients can be left alone for periods of time.

General Health

The metabolic changes induced by cancer cause the release of biologically active molecules that induce cachexia and a negative metabolic state. For some patients, metabolic steroids such as progesterone (megestrol acetate, 10 mg, once or twice a day) or corticosteroids (prednisone, 10 to 20 mg/day) may stimulate the appetite and increase the sense of well-being.

Eventually patients lose interest in food. In many ways, this is part of the natural process of death. Food should be offered, but when refused, should not be the cause of distress, divisiveness, or argument.

Although a regular diet is appropriate for some, many inactive patients prefer to eat small amounts more frequently. Custards, milk shakes, ice cream, fruit, and other snacks should be available. The American Cancer Society and the National Cancer Institute have many excellent brochures that offer suggestions to the family. Hospice teams also may have their own suggestions.

Hydration can be maintained with a variety of liquids, popsicles, and flavored ice chips. The time will come when it is difficult for the patient to swallow, and then dehydration will begin. Swabs can help maintain oral comfort for a time. The use of feeding tubes and intravenous hydration may be appropriate for some, but not to prolong a life of pain and anguish.

Pain Control

Pain in the cancer patient may be acute or chronic and may be mild, moderate, or severe. Some patients will have no pain; others may develop such severe pain that specialized pain service referrals may be required. Generally, however, the pain experienced by terminal patients can be handled well by the physician. The most important point for the physician to remember is that the patient is the authority on her own pain.

Before deciding on drug treatment, it is essential to determine the cause of the pain. A thorough pain assessment includes the history and characteristics of the pain and the physical, psychological, and spiritual status of the patient. Psychological or spiritual burdens may aggravate the physical expression of the pain. Adjunctive medications such as antidepressants as well as emotional support and counseling referrals are as important as a prescription for pain medication. Localized pain from a metastatic lesion in bone may well respond to palliative radiation therapy or splinting.

When drug therapy for pain is begun or intensified, a few general rules should be observed (Table 20-2). The drug should be selected according to the severity of the pain. The dose should be calculated according to the size and needs of the patient. For example, 60 mg of codeine will have different effects and lengths of action in 90- and 250-pound patients. The dose should be repeated before the previous dose has worn off, whether that is in 2½ or 5 hours. Regular dosing is essential because pain control is best accomplished when doses are given before the pain becomes severe.

Patients who are receiving narcotic analgesia, whether mild or strong opiates, will develop tolerance to the drug. With time, the dose will have to be increased. This is expected and acceptable.

With time, the patients also develop physical dependence on the drug, especially on the more potent opiates. This is to be expected and this too is acceptable. The physician should remember three things: (1) patients on narcotics may be particularly sensitive to the antagonist properties of mixed agonist-antagonist opiates (e.g., propoxyphene, pentazocine) and they therefore should not be used, (2) if the drugs are discontinued they must be withdrawn slowly, and (3) sudden reversal of narcotic analgesia with chemical agents (e.g., naloxone) is never necessary and is inhumane. If excessive sedation occurs, it will wear off with time, or can be reversed *slowly* by titration with a dilute solution of naloxone.

Patients may develop psychological dependence on the drug (addiction) along with physical dependence; however, the frequency of addiction is less than 1% and is acceptable if it does occur. *Under no circumstance should fear of addiction prevent adequate and humane treatment of pain in a terminally ill patient.*

The physician should not hesitate to increase the dose to continue pain control, or to select a more potent drug. Patients with chronic pain from cancer may eventually be taking hundreds of milligrams of morphine a day and yet be awake, alert, and coherent.

Worries about the potential use of drugs for suicide should be secondary to the physical comfort of the patient.

Table 20-2. Guide for pain control in the terminally ill

Determine cause of pain.
Choose appropriate drug for mild, moderate, or severe pain.
Be familiar with one or two drugs in each category.
Recognize that pain medication works best prophylactically.
Select dose according to size of the patient.
Repeat the dose according to need of the patient.
Increase the dosage or frequency as needed.
Include adjunctive medications if appropriate.
Do not worry about addiction.
Provide psychological and spiritual support as needed.

Source: Adapted from Foley KM. The treatment of cancer pain. *N Engl J Med* 313: 84–95, 1985.

Table 20-3. Drugs for pain management of mild to moderate pain

	Tabs	Frequency
Mild pain		
Acetaminophen and codeine		
325–500 mg 30–60 mg	1–2	q4h*
Ibuprofen		
600–800 mg	1	q4h
Moderate pain		
Acetaminophen and hydrocodone		
325–500 mg 5–7.5 mg	1–2	q4h*
Acetaminophen and oxycodone		
325–500 mg 5 mg	1–2	q4h*
Aspirin and oxycodone		
325–500 mg 5 mg	1–2	q4h
Oxycodone		
5 mg	1–4	q4h

*Do not exceed 4 grams per day of acetaminophen.

Mild Pain

Acetaminophen, aspirin, and the nonsteroidal antiinflammatory agents all have their place in pain management (Table 20-3). Although often combined with more potent analgesic agents, they may provide adequate control by themselves.

Combinations of acetaminophen with codeine are excellent for mild pain. Dosing is limited by limitations on the quantity of acetaminophen (more than 4 g/day results in liver toxicity) rather than limitations on the quantity of codeine.

Propoxyphene is less potent than codeine, is not to be mixed with the stronger opiates, and is not widely recommended by oncologists.

Moderate Pain

Hydrocodone and oxycodone, in combination with aspirin or acetaminophen, are excellent analgesic agents, more potent than codeine and well tolerated. Once any of the more potent narcotic analgesics are used, the physician should remember the guidelines for narcotic use (Table 20-4).

Patients may take 10 to 15 mg of hydrocodone or oxycodone at a time, but dosing is limited by the total daily dose of acetaminophen, usually when the patient requires two or more tablets every 4 hours or less. Oxycodone is available as a single agent in 5-mg tablets, which permits higher and more frequent doses without concern about the acetaminophen dose.

Narcotic drugs, especially in higher doses, produce constipation; thus, adherence to a regular program of bowel care is recommended. An example of a bowel maintenance program is provided in Table 20-5.

If patients have pain from bony metastases, nonsteroidal antiin-

Table 20-4. Guidelines for narcotic use

Choose a drug of adequate strength.
Know the pharmacology of the drug.
  preferred route of administration
  dose appropriate for route of administration
  duration of action
Adjust route and dose to patient's need.
Administer on a regular basis.
Add drugs to provide additive analgesia.
  nonsteroidal antiinflammatory drugs
Add drugs to lessen side effects.
  Dexedrine
Avoid drugs that increase sedation.
  tranquilizers
  phenothiazines
Anticipate side effects and treat.
  sedation
  nausea and vomiting
  constipation
Prevent acute withdrawal.
  Taper slowly
  never reverse sedation with full-dose naloxone

Source: Adapted from Foley KM. The treatment of cancer pain. *N Engl J Med* 313: 84–95, 1985.

Table 20-5. Bowel maintenance program

Include fruit and roughage in diet.
Take stool softeners twice a day on a regular basis.
If no bowel movement occurs for 3 days, take laxative (2 TBS milk of magnesia).
If no bowel movement occurs on morning after laxative, use bisacodyl suppository.
If no bowel movement, repeat laxative or suppository, or use disposable enema.

flammatory agents should be given around the clock because they enhance the analgesic effect of all drugs given for bone pain.

Although pentazocine is used by some physicians, it is not recommended for use. It has too many central nervous system side effects, often produces dysphoria, and should never be mixed with the stronger opiates because its antagonist properties can cause withdrawal symptoms. It is not used by oncologists.

Severe Pain

Table 20-6 lists the more commonly used drugs for treatment of severe pain. Hydromorphone, a popular street drug, is an excellent drug for oral use. It is wise, at least in some parts of the country, to warn the family not to mention that the drug is in the house.

For treatment of severe pain, *morphine* remains the drug of choice. It is now available in a wide variety of forms to facilitate its use

Table 20-6. Drugs for management of severe pain

Drug	Dose	Frequency
Hydromorphone		
Tablets (1, 2, 3, or 4 mg)	1–12 mg	q4h
Morphine sulfate		
Liquid (20 mg/ml)	10–40 mg	q2–3h
Immediate-release tablets (15–30 mg)	15–60 mg	q2–3h
Delayed-release tablets (15, 30, 60, 100 mg)	60–300 mg*	q8–12h
Fentanyl		
Transdermal patch (25, 50, 75, 100 μg/hr)	See package insert	q3 days

*Or more.

Table 20-7. Guideline for converting to morphine for increased pain control

Current pain regimen		Initial morphine dose*		
		Liquid morphine (short acting)		Timed-release tabs (long acting)
Oxycodone or hydrocodone	10 mg q4h	20 mg q3h	or	60 mg q12h
Hydromorphone	4 mg q4h	20 mg q3h	or	60 mg q12h
	8 mg q4h	40 mg q3h	or	120 mg q12h

*Continue acetaminophen or nonsteroidal antiinflammatory drugs.

outside of the hospital: liquid or tablets for oral administration, as well as wax-based tablets for prolonged duration of action. By judicious use of combinations of these forms, most patients can remain pain-free. Table 20-7 provides a guideline for changing patients from one type of pain medication to morphine. The somnolence produced by morphine usually disappears in a few days and patients remain amazingly alert.

The oral preparations have about one-third the potency of parenteral morphine: 30 mg of oral morphine would be equal to 10 mg given parenterally.

If the patient has intermittent severe pain, for example, when having a dressing change or when getting into a bath tub, 10 to 20 mg of liquid morphine can be given. Its onset of action will begin in 5 or 10 minutes and will last for 2 to 3 hours. If the patient begins to need frequent doses of morphine, she can be switched to the long-acting form. For example, if the patient requires nine doses of 20 mg in a 24-hour period, the 180-mg daily dose can be divided into two or three doses and given in the long-acting preparation: 90 mg every 12 hours or 60 mg every 8 hours. The long-acting preparation has its onset of action in 4 hours, but lasts for 8 to 12. Once the patient has around-the-clock pain control from the long-acting morphine, small intermittent doses of the liquid short-acting drug can be used for breakthrough pain.

If the patient cannot take oral medication, several other options are available. A central venous access device can be inserted and continuous infusions of morphine given via a small electronically controlled pump. In switching to parenteral dosing, the total daily dosage of oral morphine is calculated, divided by 3 to obtain the parenteral equivalence, and divided by the 24 hours of the day to obtain the dosage per hour that can be delivered via the infusion pump. Morphine can be given rectally; this is as effective as oral administration. In patients unable to take oral or rectal opioid analgesics, the subcutaneous route may be used. Intramuscular dosing should never be used because of the difficulty in administering an injection to a cachectic patient and the pain of the injection.

Fentanyl, an opioid analgesic usually used for anesthesia, is now available in a transdermal preparation that can provide continuous pain control. Many patients, however, experience dysphoria with this drug. It is difficult to titrate doses because of its long-acting effects. In general, it should not be used in combination with morphine except by physicians very well versed in pain management.

Adjuvant Drug Therapy

Adjuvant drugs, which are not analgesics, can be used to treat specific problems or types of pain. They are not prescribed routinely but only for specific purposes. Examples are shown in Table 20-8.

Table 20-8. Adjuvant drugs for pain control

Indication	Drug	Dose[a,b]
Depression	Amitriptyline	25–100 mg at bedtime
Anxiety	Diazepam	5–10 mg q8–12h
	Lorazepam	0.5–2.0 mg q8–12h
	Chlorpromazine	10–25 mg q4–8h
	Dronabinol	2.5–5.0 mg q4–6h
Agitation, psychosis	Chlorpromazine	10–25 mg q4–8h
	Haloperidol	1–10 mg q8–12h
Neuritic pain	Phenytoin	100–300 mg/day
	Carbamazepine	100–400 mg/day
	Amitriptyline	25–75 mg/day
Antiinflammatory	Prednisone	10–60 mg/day
Cord compression	Dexamethasone	16–64 mg/day
Intracranial pressure	Dexamethasone	16–64 mg/day
Appetite stimulation	Prednisone	10–20 mg/day
	Megestrol	10–20 mg/day
	Dronabinol	2.5–5.0 mg q4h

[a]Start at lowest dose and increase to desired effect.
[b]All doses administered PO.

Depression is common and can be treated with amitriptyline, a drug that is also useful to potentiate narcotics and to treat dysesthetic pain. Anxiolytics, such as diazepam or lorazepam, are helpful for panic attacks or acute anxiety, as can be chlorpromazine. Dronabinol (the active ingredient of marijuana) can be helpful but some patients do not like the psychic effects. Neuroleptic drugs such as chlorpromazine and haloperidol may be helpful if severe agitation is preventing adequate pain control. Sedation, however, can be a problem. Anticonvulsants such as phenytoin suppress spontaneous neuronal firing and can be helpful when used in conjunction with, but not in place of, narcotics for neuritic pain such as trigeminal neuralgia or nerve root pain. The antiinflammatory properties of prednisone and dexamethasone can be a benefit in nerve or spinal cord compression and in the treatment of increased intracranial pressure. They also stimulate appetite and feelings of well-being. Progesterone and dronabinol also aid in appetite stimulation.

Special Circumstances

In special circumstances when pain is not controlled with parenteral drugs, epidural or intraventricular catheters can be placed for the infusion of morphine directly into the central nervous system. This may be helpful for those patients who require enormous doses of morphine every day or are too somnolent. By infusing the drug directly adjacent to the pain fibers, much lower doses are required. To avoid acute withdrawal and seizures when changing to epidural or intraventricular dosing, extreme care must be taken to withdraw the patient slowly and carefully from the high systemic doses.

Anesthesiologists and neurosurgeons can perform ablative procedures for patients with severe regional pain problems and may be consulted for special pain problems.

Suggested Reading

Palliative Care

Doyle D, Hanks GWC, and Macdonald N, eds. Oxford Textbook of Palliative Medicine. Oxford: Oxford University Press, 1993.

Higginson I, Wade A, and McCarthy M. Palliative care: Views of patients and their families. *Br Med J* 301:277–280, 1990.

Porzsolt F, and Tannock I. Goals of palliative cancer therapy. *J Clin Oncol* 11:378–381, 1993.

Slevin ML. Quality of life: Philosophical question or clinical reality? *Br Med J* 305:466–469, 1992.

Pain Control

Foley KM. The treatment of cancer pain. *N Engl J Med* 313:84–95, 1985.

Hill CS. The barriers to adequate pain management with opioid analgesics. *Sem Oncol* 20(suppl):1–5, 1993.

Portenoy RK. Cancer pain: Pathophysiology and syndromes. *Lancet* 339:1026–1036, 1992.

Portenoy RK. Cancer pain management. *Sem Oncol* 20(suppl):19–35, 1993.

World Health Organization. *Cancer Pain Relief.* Geneva, 1986.

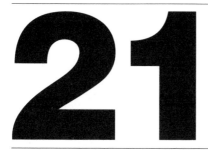

Psychosocial Issues

Margaret Deanesly

The female breast is a unique appendage. It is a talisman of sexuality to the woman and an erotic delight for the woman and her partner. It is a dynamic, endocrine-responsive functional unit whose size and sensations ebb and flow with each menstrual cycle. The breast is the quintessential bonding unit and succor of the infant.

Any cosmetic distortion of the breast brings with it disruption of many aspects of self-image, self-esteem, and wholeness. The doctor who, with a specially trained nurse or assistant, is prepared to answer the myriad nonsurgical questions of a woman facing breast surgery will greatly enhance and speed the psychosocial recovery of these patients.

Perisurgical Distress Reactions

Breast surgery is both a physical and an emotional assault on feelings of femininity and sexuality. Patients are initially caught up in the root worry that this illness may spell death, and are working out optimal treatment plans with several consultants. It is not until the breast is gone or disfigured that the grief of loss may express itself. Feeling that they have coped well through the surgical phase of care the patient is surprised to find herself depressed and mourning at a time when she thought the worst was over. The well-known sequence of denial, anger, and sadness followed by acceptance may have been delayed by the early coping mechanisms around the surgery. This late distress often comes several months after diagnosis and initial treatment. It should be anticipated by the doctor and watched for by trained staff or forewarned family members.

A recent study of the psychosocial responses of women to breast surgery found wide variety in the depth and manifestations of psychosocial problems as well as in their timing. The study found that women who were emotionally intact and mature prior to surgery did best. A history of psychological maladaptation to pregnancy, menses, or marriage may forewarn the primary care giver that more intervention and time need to be taken with a particular patient. Even the most poised and able women, however, may find the double threats of disfigurement and death daunting prospects. It is incumbent upon the primary care physician, or the doctor who sees the

Table 21-1. Questions to unmask depression

How are you sleeping? What time do you waken?
How's your appetite? Does food taste good?
Are you moody or frightened?
Have you cried about having breast cancer?
Do you laugh and experience joy again?
Are you back to work yet?
How's your wardrobe coming along? Have you bought a prosthesis yet?
Have you and your lover resumed intercourse? Why not?
What are your plans for the future?

patient and family frequently, to alert the patient to the emotional component of breast cancer and to provide reassurance that she will heal emotionally as well as physically. The patient should be referred to supportive care groups as needed.

Evidence of depression may be masked as the patient tries to be cheery and "good." The true nature of the patient's mood will only reveal itself if time is taken to listen in a nonjudgmental fashion with an ear attuned to the typical manifestations of depression (Table 21-1). The patient first must come to grips with the life-threatening aspects of her diagnosis. Only then can she begin to take other steps necessary to mourn her loss. Every effort should be made to encourage the expression of feelings of anger, sadness, fear, and grief by counseling, inquiry, and psychiatric or group counseling referral if necessary.

Late or Delayed Postsurgical Reactions

Some patients will not show any adverse psychological symptoms after mastectomy. It is unlikely that this is the healthy sign that both the patient and doctor wish it to be. Delayed reactions may manifest themselves many months or years later if an unwanted major life change such as a family death or divorce robs the patient of her last vestiges of self-denial, compensatory coping mechanisms, or ego strength. In a delayed reaction, the cause of her unexpected depression or personality change may be difficult to ferret out and resistant to treatment. Often, a thorough and intimate discussion of her feelings about her malignancy and how it has affected her personal life will unearth these underlying currents of distress. It is never easy to ask a patient specific questions about intercourse, petting, nude behavior, or fantasy life, but until such issues are inquired about the patient may be unable to speak of them. These questions give patients the "permission" to have these feelings, to speak of them, and to get answers to questions they dared not ask before. It is not unusual to unearth a great deal of psychosexual dysfunction

Table 21-2. Psychosexual dysfunction: appropriate and inappropriate questions

Appropriate	Inappropriate
Are you and your partner comfortable with hugging, petting, and cuddling?	How's your sex life?
Are you finding comfortable positions for intercourse?	How's your sex life?
What parts of your life are different now than they were before your surgery?	How are you doing, dear?
Tell me about your sleeping. What time do you go to bed? What time do you waken? Do you sleep the whole night without wakening and waken rested?	You sleeping OK?
What brand of prosthesis have you decided on?	Are you doing OK with clothing?
At your next visit, I want you to bring your swimsuit and model it for my nurse and me.	You may need a new swimsuit to cover this scar.
What questions do you have? Which support group have you joined?	Here's a pamphlet about your disease. Some people like support groups.

on the part of the patient or her mate in these interviews. Table 21-2 suggests appropriate and inappropriate questions to ask. Remember that her "I'm OK" and his curt "just fine" may be cover-ups and should, despite their uneasiness, prompt you to continue probing in order to drain this festering emotional wound.

Sources of Help

Having identified psychological distress that seems to be delaying your patient's recovery, you must decide whether referral is necessary. As a general rule, patients still in trouble 6 months or more after surgery will need fairly sophisticated and time-consuming help. The cheapest and often the best help comes from breast cancer support groups. If the patient cannot be persuaded to attend such a meeting or none is available in her community, the nearest American Cancer Society or even a prosthesis fitter may be able to refer the patient to a counselor who specializes in these cases. Because treatment usually consists of allowing the patient to vent her feelings in a safe setting, a clinical psychologist or marriage counselor often does very well. Referring the patient to her pastor, rabbi, or other religious figure sometimes can be sufficient *if that is the patient's choice.*

This chapter chronicles the physical, social, and sexual hurdles women and their partners face from the time a lump is discovered until full posttreatment rehabilitation is attained. Its purpose is to provide breast physicians and their nurses with practical information germane to all breast illness cases.

Finding the Lump

Whether found on self-examination or by physician or radiologic examination the awareness of a breast lump strikes *terror* into the heart of the woman. This cloud of fear will complicate all interviews and attempts to instruct the patient. The style of the doctor-patient relationship established during the case work-up will greatly influence the outcome of the myriad psychosocial issues that inevitably arise. This needs to be kept uppermost in the minds of the care givers if cooperation and a constructive doctor-patient team are to be created.

Early Diagnostic Phase

The more expeditious and efficient a breast lump work-up is, the better for the patient. While waiting for the final word on the benign or malignant nature of the mass, the patient is distraught and her mind is a jumble of "what if's." Hopefully she has shared her concerns with a loved one, and he or she is equally caught up in these fears. The sensitivity of the radiology technicians, the doctor's personnel, and physicians to the fragile psyche of these women sets the tone for the next phase of care.

These women need to feel that they can ask questions, repeatedly if necessary, at all stages of their care and of all care givers. Answers need to be direct, complete, and devoid of medical jargon. It is not unusual for patients to become disturbed when they hear what seems to them to be conflicting answers to their questions. Time spent patiently and lovingly explaining will help. Many women will repeat the same questions over and over. Written information dispensed during the early diagnostic phase can help if it is not too complex. Because the diagnosis is not yet made, this is not the time to use a pamphlet that talks about the fine points of management or the side effects of chemotherapy.

Presenting the Diagnosis of Breast Cancer

Women should ideally hear the dreaded diagnosis of breast cancer in the company of an understanding loved one. Doctors need to schedule plenty of time for tears and to present options for treatment. Women usually are sufficiently distraught that repetition of information is essential. A written sheet explaining care options can be helpful and in some states such a disclosure sheet is required by law. Encouraging patients to bring in written questions can improve initial exchanges of information. The use by the patient of a simple cassette tape recorder during office visits allows her to review questions, answers, and advice at home and with others.

Patients should be informed of how long they have to make up their minds about care options. Most centers show no degradation of outcome with up to a 3-week interval between diagnosis and definitive care. The longer the waiting period, however, the more indecision and confusing anecdotal advice may plague the patient and her family.

While women seem to do better emotionally if they take charge of their care and feel that they can influence that care, most are ill-equipped to make sophisticated clinical decisions. The careful teaching of the anatomy, vocabulary, and options of management are of primary importance in helping women make decisions. A specially trained registered nurse or physician's assistant can help greatly with this education.

Involving the patient in self-education and making her a member of the team that is being marshaled to provide her care is essential. This involvement will benefit the patient by making her feel empowered instead of impoverished or "like just one more breast." The doctor will be rewarded with a helpful rather than hindering patient as the complex demands on her mental, physical, and emotional coping skills arise. With this style of care patients feel listened to, cared about, and joined in their struggle.

The time of presentation of the diagnosis is often the time to begin forming the care team. This is also the time to encourage the patient to seek a second opinion. Many patients are reluctant to ask for a second opinion for fear that it will be read by the physician as a lack of confidence or, worse yet, as an insult. Many think that this presumed slight will negatively affect their care.

Now is the time to let the patient and her family know that everything possible is being done for her physical and emotional well-being. Introducing the patient to a radiation oncologist or an oncologist specializing in breast cancer care at this time will get many questions answered. These time-consuming interviews are time well spent. A registered nurse or social worker readily available by phone and specially trained in this field can be an invaluable resource for the patient and a major physician time-saver.

Immediate Postsurgical Psychosocial Problems

Except in cases of needle biopsy, women begin the emotional healing process by accepting scarring and local discomfort of the breast postoperatively. That breast will never be the same and its appearance will be a constant reminder of her neoplasia to both her and her partner. Table 21-3 presents some do's and dont's to consider in the management of the patient.

A scar that looks tiny to the physician may look larger and more disfiguring to the patient. The physician's knowledge of how scars age, change, and fade may allow him or her to overlook angry redness or minor lumps that will flatten, and to disregard transient pares-

Table 21-3. Guiding patient adjustment to the postsurgical breast

Appropriate	Inappropriate
Open-ended appointment	Fixed "12-minute" encounter
Nonjudgmental listening	Quick-fix answers to concerns and questions
Information about scar appearance at each stage of healing	"Looks great!"
Have the loved one present at follow-up and dressing changes	Distract patient from looking at healing
Overdo kindness, reassurance, encouragement, and understanding	Impersonal "automatic care"
Provide knowledgeable references for prostheses fitters	Allow patient to find clothing and prostheses purveyors on her own

thesias. These distortions, however, may be a major concern to the patient. Explanations about the stages of healing and everlasting reassurance avoid later pathological reactions. Telling a woman her mastectomy or scar "looks wonderful" will only alienate the physician from her at a time when she needs help the most. The expressions "healing normally," "doing fine," or "just like it should be at this stage," often relieve some anxiety. Downplaying the family's revulsion, horror, or fear will not be constructive. Patients and families have a completely different frame of reference than the physician does in this matter. Not only have they probably never seen surgical scarring before, but it is *their* minds and bodies that are hurting with a problem that will not go away.

Patients and their partners often are frightened or revolted by the appearance of the surgical sight. Explaining the shape, texture, and color of scarring during dressing changes helps. Reassurance about normal healing stages speeds acceptance.

The Pros and Cons of Reconstruction

For some women, breast reconstruction at the time of primary surgery or soon thereafter is essential for emotional rehabilitation. For others prolonged or repeat surgery is an anathema. Results of reconstruction, while often excellent, do not produce a mass that feels or functions as a breast. The value of the reconstructed breast is largely in the eye of the beholder; it may be of great or little importance depending on the individual patient. For some women, how they look to others, especially men, is paramount. Patients need to see photographs of real reconstructions, not just of the best outcomes but typical outcomes as well. Ideally they should speak to other patients who are reconstructed as well as to some who opted not to undergo reconstruction prior to making their decision.

Many women do not realize that a reconstructed breast that looks perfect in clothing may look peculiar in night clothes or in the nude. The appearance, texture, and feel of the nude reconstructed breast may be displeasing to the patient or her partner. No woman wants it to be obvious to one who casually hugs her that one breast is hard and the other soft, as can happen with some procedures. The relative absence of erotic sensations in the reconstructed breast may be an unthought of issue and deserves to be raised before surgery rather than coped with afterward.

Most surgical reconstructions avoid the need for external removable pads and allow the patient to appear clothed as she did prior to surgery. The latest external, removable prostheses are so lifelike and adaptable that they are fully satisfactory to most older, emotionally stable women. External prostheses can be glued onto the body for days at a time or stuffed into a myriad of lacy garments for any and all clothed activities without fear of the prosthesis being dislodged or identified.

Sex Partners, Absent Breasts, and Libido

Most men interviewed after their wife's mastectomy admit few sexual problems as a result of the disfigurement of the partner's chest. Fear of causing discomfort in the healing surgical site can be a transient problem but erotic satisfaction remains adequate. Patients dearly need their partner's reassurance about this initially. Nonbreast sexual activity assumes greater importance in the postsurgical patient. Hugs, massages, showering together, and all forms of petting and erotica acceptable to both partners should be encouraged.

A crude advertising adage summarizes the problems faced by the woman with a surgically disfigured breast: "Tits sell beer." The constant barrage of breast nudity, cleavage, and symmetrical torso curvature on magazine covers, billboards, and movie screens is an acid reminder to the patient of what she has lost. Concealed surgical losses of other body parts, such as the colon, lung, or thyroid, do not elicit these problems, largely because these organs are devoid of sexual connotation and are not constantly foisted into the public eye. Quite literally, their removal is not titillating. Remembering that the breast is more than just another organ will provide the perspective that a physician needs to promote total emotional and physical healing.

Changed libido on the part of the patient or her partner is multifactorial. Disfigurement, discomfort, and depression all contribute to changed sexual responsiveness. The side effects of adjuvant therapy or fatigue resulting from radiation treatments may contribute to decreased frequency of intercourse. Adjuvant therapy itself may decrease the female libido and may contribute to low estrogen symptoms of dyspareunia and vaginal dryness.

Sexual Intercourse

Sexual intercourse can be resumed as soon as the patient is comfortable. This normal activity can be psychosexually therapeutic. Patients may need some suggestions for comfortable intercourse positions. Experimentation works best, but you can get the ball rolling by suggesting that the woman be on top, that coitus can take place in recliner chairs, hot tubs or pools, or in any fashion that initially, at least, does not require the surgical site to bear the full weight or friction of the partner's body. Patients in "missionary position" can be instructed to place the affected arm across the chest with the hand on the opposite shoulder to create a protective bridge over the surgical site or to cover the surgery with a small crib-sized pillow until she is without discomfort. Partners need to be reassured that normal sexual activity will cause no harm.

Women often will want to wear a "rest breast" or a light prosthesis with her night clothes until she is comfortable and used to her scarring. Now is the time for treating the patient to new, indulgent sexy lingerie, preferably bought by or with the spouse or lover.

Few patients or mates will ask the "When can we?" question. Doctors need to suggest, remind, or even assign sexual intercourse as a healing activity.

Bras and Clothing

As soon as the patient is able to dress, cheap, simple adjustments can be made to bras and clothing. A normal, symmetrical breast appearance is a tonic to the postsurgical patient. Soft, clean cotton stuffed into a section of old nylon stocking makes a light false breast to place in the bra cavity. The clips that control the length of bra straps should be posterior and over the scapulae. Bras with front clips may cause chafing of the surgical area.

Until the vacant bra cup is filled with something, clothing will not drape properly, and patients may be reluctant to be seen in public. A soft stuffed bra can usually be worn by the tenth postoperative day.

Prostheses

Women with modified radical mastectomies or more than 30% removal of breast tissue will need something similar in texture and weight to normal breast tissue to fill the vacant bra cup after full healing has taken place.

Breast reconstruction may serve this purpose. In the absence of reconstruction, the surgeon or his or her designee can become knowledgeable about local sources of bras, expert fitters, and prostheses. A phone call to the American Cancer Society will establish where these businesses are (see Appendix C). Most surgical supply houses carry prostheses but they are often not very pleasant places to get help, surrounded as one will be by bedpans, wheelchairs, and all manner of replacement parts and sickroom supplies. At surgical conventions and educational meetings at which breast cancer is discussed, it is common to see several booths purveying prostheses with hand-out literature and samples to feel and compare. Doctors should become familiar with these products. Several mail-order companies exist and have product catalogs. Most major urban department stores have a brassiere fitter (who may or may not have special training) in the lingerie department, but the store may be limited to one brand or style. In metropolitan areas, boutiques devoted to the unique clothing needs of breast surgical patients, including lingerie, swimwear, and pocketed bras are appearing. While often more expensive than mail-order catalogs or department stores for the often distressing initial fitting, they can be guaranteed to provide the patient with knowledgeable and supportive service.

Bras come with and without pockets. Prostheses are made with and without nipples. Much trial and error in the first 6 months after surgery is needed before a comfortable and attractive fit is obtained. Patients should be advised to buy one bra at a time. Many stores will allow prostheses to be taken on a trial basis. Some insurance plans will cover these costs if the doctor prescribes the prosthesis and the shop receipt notes "surgical prosthesis." A "lingerie" receipt is not sufficient for claim. In 1993, most prostheses cost between $250 and $400. With normal wear and gentle care they last at least a year. Changes in body weight of about 10 pounds or more necessitate a new fitting.

The fitting of the first postoperative bra and prosthesis is emotionally very taxing. Ideally, patients should not go alone. Staring at the nude scarred chest is inevitable and brings home the permanence of the deformity.

During the 6-week or 3-month postoperative office visit, the surgeon or his or her nurse should discuss the cosmetic adjustments of the patient. Patients need to feel that they can be embraced without having the prosthesis detected. Adjustments to swimwear and lingerie should be inquired about. The active sportswoman must feel secure that her external silicone breast will not shift and embarrass her while jogging, bowling, playing tennis, or any other sport.

Some women prefer to wear their prosthesis in a light lacy bra in bed at night. The larger the remaining breast, the more necessary this is for shoulder comfort. A soft mattress or water bed that conforms to the body and fills in the space left by breast removal makes this practice unnecessary.

Adjuvant Therapy and Psychological Recovery

The need for adjuvant therapy prolongs the acute phase of breast cancer illness. While some women have little trouble, most have periods of illness, prolonged morbid thoughts, and a protracted adjustment to a positive outlook.

Some chemotherapy further complicates body image and self-esteem by causing hair loss. A pretreatment wig fitting can ease this transition with hair pieces designed to mimic the hair before its thinning or loss. Women can be assured that hair will regrow.

Antiestrogen treatment may lead to dyspareunia secondary to vaginal dryness and vulvar atrophy. Topical applications of nonestrogenic moisturizers will improve vulvovaginal lubrication. It may be necessary to use water-soluble lubricants at the time of intercourse. Antiestrogens also can result in a change in the size of the remaining breast tissue, necessitating a refitting of the prosthesis.

The Role of the Support Group

Postmastectomy support groups abound. At the time of surgery, doctors can arrange for visitation of their patients in the hospital by American Cancer Society Reach to Recover volunteers. The volunteers are women with breast cancer (at least 1 year postoperatively) who bring role-model support, information, and a kit that contains a temporary bra-stuffing form. Once at home, patients can request this service from the ACS without a doctor's order.

Ongoing, long-term support groups, especially for those undergoing chemotherapy, are of tremendous value. One study even showed an increase in survival time of those attending such a group. Women feel at ease and share hopes, fears, coping mechanisms, and information. These groups can be located through other patients, hospitals, or the American Cancer Society.

The public library and specialized lay medical libraries shelve much written material about breast cancer. Some is professionally written, other is biographical, anecdotal, or simplified. Some patients are helped by extensive reading while others are frightened; reading recommendations need to be tailored accordingly.

Summary

The surgeon and his or her staff are encouraged to treat the mind of the breast cancer patient with the same detail and care that they give to the surgical site. Such attention will speed the patient's recovery and enhance the patient's emotional well-being.

Suggested Reading

Coscarelli-Schag CA, et al. Characteristics of women at risk for psychosocial distress in the year after breast cancer. *J Clin Oncol* 11: 783–793, 1993.

Schain WS, and Fetting JH. Modified radical mastectomy versus breast conservation: Psychosocial considerations. *Sem Oncol* 19: 239–243, 1992.

Appendixes

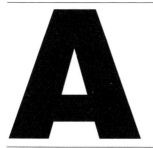

Breast Self-Examination

Lois F. O'Grady

Breast self-examination (BSE) is an integral part of the breast health program for two reasons. First, 10% to 15% of cancers do not show up on mammograms. And second, among populations of women who do not have routine mammography, the majority of tumors are detected by the patient herself. This appendix is designed to instruct the clinician in those BSE techniques that are most easily taught, retained, and practiced by the lay public.

All women over the age of 20 should be instructed in BSE, and the teaching should be reviewed periodically so that by the time the woman is in the high-risk years, she is both adept at and comfortable with the procedure. To help physicians and patients, the American Cancer Society (ACS) has developed helpful leaflets that contain detailed instructions for BSE. These are available at no cost as a public service of the ACS. A supply for your office may be obtained by calling your local unit of the American Cancer Society, or by calling 1-800-ACS-2345.

The text and figures presented below are adapted with permission from the American Cancer Society, California Division, Inc., leaflet entitled "Breast Self-Examination: A New Approach," code #6438.39, dated 5/92.

General Information

Women should examine their breasts 5 to 7 days after the onset of menses each month. At this time, the breasts are the least swollen and the least tender. Menopausal women should select a specific monthly date, for example, the first, for their monthly examination. Women who have augmented breasts should continue to perform BSE as should pregnant women. Nursing women can examine their breasts after all milk has been expressed. In these latter groups, the examination will not be as sensitive, but it is better than no examination at all.

Patients need to learn the following:

1. Correct positions
2. Area to be examined
3. Palpation technique
4. Pattern of search
5. Nipple examination
6. Axillary examination

Positions

Inspection

Figure A-1 shows the four positions used for visual inspection of the breast. While standing, look for changes in contour and shape of the breasts, color and texture of the skin and nipple, and evidence of nipple discharge. Standing in a well-lighted room before a mirror, the patient performs the inspection with arms relaxed at the side (A), hands on the hips (B), arms raised above the head (C), and bending forward (D).

Palpation

The woman will palpate her breasts while lying in one of two positions: lying flat or lying partially on the side. The former is best for women with small breasts, the latter for women with larger breasts because it is a better position for stretching the breast out along the chest wall and facilitating palpation of the lateral quadrants.

The opposite hand will be used to palpate the breast: left hand for right breast, and right hand for left breast.

Lying Flat

This position is shown in Fig. A-2. The woman lies flat on her back with a small pillow or folded towel under the shoulder of the breast to be examined.

Lying to the Side

In this position (Fig. A-3), the woman lies on the side opposite the breast to be examined, left side to examine right breast. She then rotates her torso so that the shoulders are flat, and the arm on the side of the breast to be examined is placed over the head. A pillow or towel is not used.

Area to Be Examined

The area to be examined (Fig. A-4), for each breast, extends from the midsternal line to the midaxillary line, and from the clavicle to a line drawn 1 to 2 inches below the inframammary fold. The woman should be advised of the axillary tail, that portion of the breast which extends toward the axilla. This area and the rest of the upper outer quadrant contains more breast tissue than the other quadrants and merits special attention.

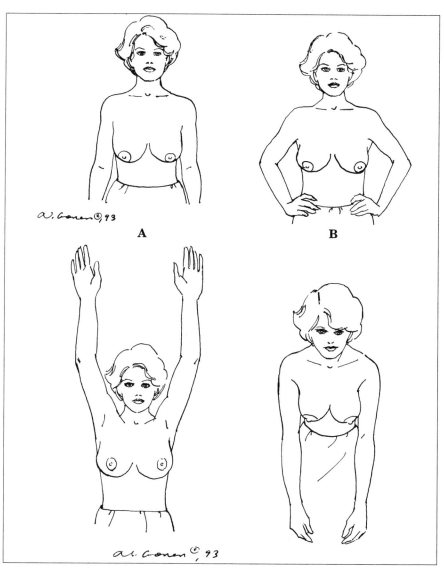

Fig. A-1. The positions for visual inspection of the breasts: A. arms relaxed at the side; B. hands on hips; C. arms raised above the head; and D. bending forward.

Palpation Technique

Palpation is performed with the pads of three or four fingers (Fig. A-5). The woman is instructed to move the fingers in continuous circles, about the size of a dime, passing the breast tissue between her fingers and the chest wall. Each circle should be done with both light and firm palpation. The palpating fingers are never lifted. Lotion or

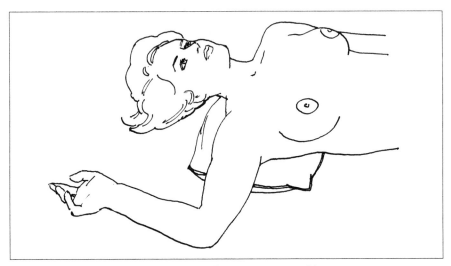

Fig. A-2. Position for palpation of small to average-sized breasts.

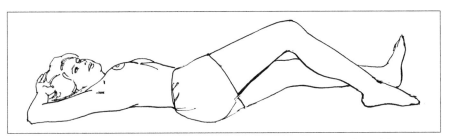

Fig. A-3. Position for palpation of large breasts. This exaggerated position stretches the breast across a wider area for ease of palpation.

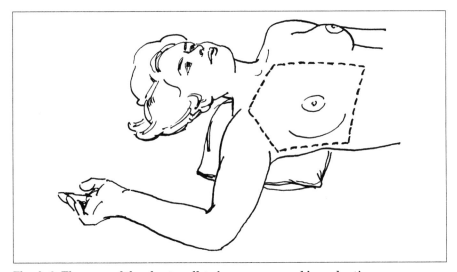

Fig. A-4. The area of the chest wall to be encompassed by palpation.

talcum powder may be used to facilitate the sliding motion of the fingers over the skin.

Pattern of Search

Three patterns of search are popular. The woman should select the one she likes best and use it exclusively. Some women need a reminder to examine beneath the nipple-areolar complex.

Circular

In this technique, the breast is imagined to be the face of a clock and palpated at each "hour" in concentric circles until the entire area is covered (Fig. A-6). Eight to ten circles may need to be made.

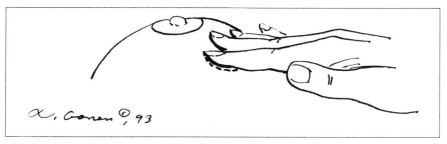

Fig. A-5. The proper position of the fingers for palpation.

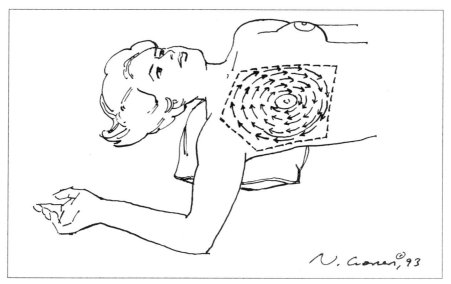

Fig. A-6. The circular pattern for palpation. This pattern is preferred by many health practitioners.

Although this is the classic technique performed by health professionals, many women find the vertical strip technique easier.

Vertical Strip

Starting in the axilla or at the sternal line (Fig. A-7), the rotary palpation is performed in longitudinal strips about one-finger breadth in width. This usually means four strips between the sternal line and the nipple and six between the nipple and midaxillary line. Larger women may need more.

Wheel Spokes

Figure A-8 shows the wheel-spokes pattern. The technique is the same as in the vertical strip pattern.

Nipple Examination

After palpation, each nipple should be squeezed gently to see if there is any change (Fig. A-9). Some women never have a discharge, some have intermittent discharge, and some have continuous discharge. A change in pattern, color, or frequency of discharge may be significant.

Axillary Examination

With the arm relaxed at the side (Fig. A-10), the axilla can be palpated. The fingers of the examining hand are placed high in the axilla and swept downward, compressing the axillary contents between the fingers and the chest wall.

Reinforcement

Figure A-11 reminds each of us that clinical examination of the breast is part of the basic health examination. It provides an opportunity to reinforce the importance of BSE and to review the technique used by the patient.

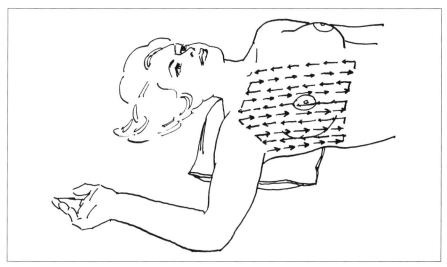

Fig. A-7. The vertical strip pattern for palpation. Many patients find this technique easier than the circular pattern.

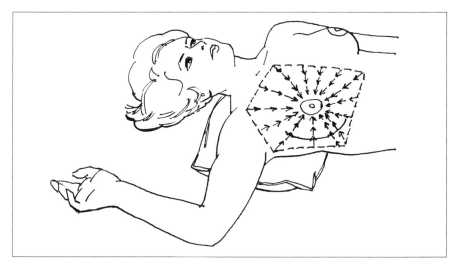

Fig. A-8. The wheel spokes pattern for palpation.

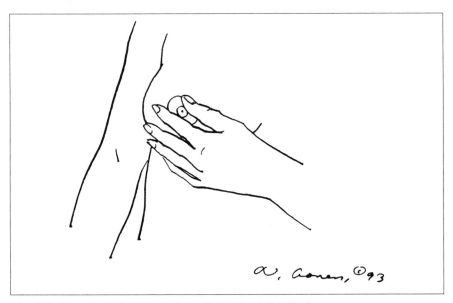

Fig. A-9. The nipple is squeezed gently to check for discharge.

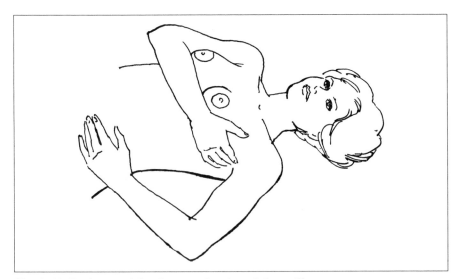

Fig. A-10. Patient position for examination of the axillae.

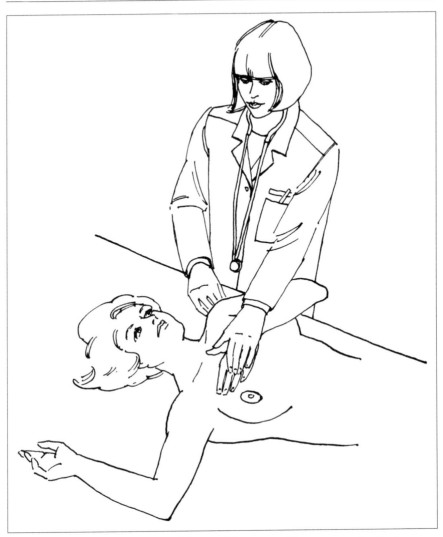

Fig. A-11. Examination by a health practitioner provides an opportunity to teach or reinforce breast self-examination techniques.

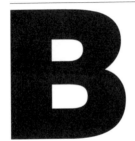

Breast Health History Form

University of California, Davis
Medical Center

Breast Health History

Date of Exam _____

YOUR NAME _____

AGE _____

NAME OF YOUR DOCTOR _____

HAVE YOU HAD A MAMMOGRAM BEFORE? Yes ☐ No ☐
If yes, where was it done? _____ and
How long ago? _____

DO YOU HAVE ANY MEDICAL PROBLEMS WITH YOUR BREASTS? Yes ☐ No ☐
If yes, please explain _____
_____

DO YOU OR YOUR DOCTOR FEEL A LUMP IN YOUR BREASTS? Yes ☐ No ☐
If yes, where? _____
How long has it been there? _____

DO YOU HAVE A HISTORY OF BREAST CANCER? Yes ☐ No ☐
If yes, did you have ☐ Radiation Therapy? or ☐ chemotherapy?

HAVE YOU HAD PREVIOUS BREAST SURGERY OR BIOPSY? Yes ☐ No ☐
If yes, which side was it done on? Right ☐ Left ☐
Explain what was done _____
_____
When was it done? _____(year)
What was found? _____

HAS ANY BLOOD RELATIVE HAD BREAST CANCER? Yes ☐ No ☐
If yes, which relative?_____

ARE YOU STILL HAVING MENSTRUAL PERIODS? Yes ☐ No ☐
When was your last period? _____

DO YOU TAKE HORMONES? Yes ☐ No ☐
If yes, what type? _____ How long? _____

IS THERE ANY OTHER INFORMATION THAT WOULD BE HELPFUL FOR US TO KNOW?
_____
_____
_____

THANK YOU

LEFT   RIGHT

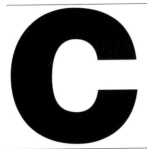

Support Groups and Equipment Suppliers

Resources

The American Cancer Society
In most communities, the American Cancer Society (ACS) provides the following services: information and counseling; loans of sickroom supplies, comfort items, and surgical dressings; transportation to and from treatments; and medical assistance for all cancer patients. The valuable program "I can cope" is sponsored through the ACS. Phone: 1-800-ACS-2345.

Breast Cancer Advisory Center, Inc.
Box 224
Kensington, MD 20895
Nonprofit group designed to provide information on all aspects of breast cancer.

Cancer Information Service
National Cancer Institute
1-800-4-CANCER

The Komen Alliance
3500 Gaston Ave
Baylor University Medical Center
Dallas, TX 75246
A program for the research and treatment of breast disease. Also available at 1-800-462-9273 is the Susan G. Komen Foundation, 6820 LBJ Freeway, Suite 130, Dallas, TX 75240.

Make Today Count
P.O. Box 22
Osage Beach, MO 65065
A nonprofit organization for cancer patients and their families.

National Cancer Institute (NCI)
Office of Cancer Communications
Bethesda, MD 20892

National Coalition for Cancer Survivorship
323 Eight Street, NW
Albuquerque, NM 87102
505-764-9956
The goal of this national group is to generate a nationwide awareness of survivorship, showing that people live quality lives after
cancer.

The National Hospice Organization
1901 North Fort Meyer Drive
Suite 307
Arlington, VA 22209
703-243-5900
This organization acts as a clearinghouse for over 1000 hospices
throughout the country.

National Lymphedema Network
2215 Post Street
San Francisco, CA 94115
1-800-541-3259
This nonprofit organization was founded to meet the informational
and treatment needs of people who suffer from lymphedema.

RENU (Reconstructive Education for National Understanding)
A division of the Einstein Medical Center in Philadelphia that offers
a hot-line counseling service for women considering breast reconstruction. Phone: 215-456-7383.

Support Group Programs

YWCA Encore
Contact YWCA National Headquarters
726 Broadway
New York, NY 10003
212-614-2827
A support group and aquatic exercise program where one "does not
need to know how to swim, and your hair will stay dry." Provides
therapeutic water exercises to increase flexibility and restore full
range of motion to the axilla and pectoral muscles. (Note: Not all
YWCAs offer Encore.)

Y-ME Breast Cancer Support Program
18220 Harwood Avenue
Homewood, IL 60430
1-800-221-2141 or 312-799-8228
This self-help program, started by breast cancer patients, confronts
the challenges faced by newly diagnosed women. Branches are
nationwide.

Look Good, Feel Better

A program of the American Cancer Society. Trained community volunteers skilled in the application of cosmetics, hair and wig design, and fashion assist members to improve their self-image and appearance. Call the nearest American Cancer Society or the national office: Tower Place, 3340 Peachtree Road, NE, Atlanta, GA 30026. Phone: 1-800-ACS-2345.

Equipment for Lymphedema Therapy

Bio-Compression Systems, Inc.
736 Gotham Parkway
Carlstadt, NJ 07072
1-800-888-0908

Camp, International
P.O. Box 89
Jackson, MI 49204
1-800-492-1088

JOBST
P.O. Box 653
Toledo, OH 43694
1-419-698-1611

Wright-Linear
2211 Post Street, Suite 404
San Francisco, CA 94115
1-800-541-3259

Manual Lymph Drainage
1-800-642-2046

National Lymphedema Network
1-800-541-3259

Index

Index

616.
994
49
PRA

5000592120

CL
616.
994
49
PRA